7 Laws Of Getting Lean

G000123203

by Joe Warner and Jon Lipsey

Art Editor Ian Ferguson
Photography Glen Burrows
Model Jaimie-Beth Geraghty
Managing Editor Chris Miller
Additional Photography iStock

Publisher Steven O'Hara
Publishing Director Dan Savage
Marketing Manager Charlotte Park
Commercial Director Nigel Hole

Printed by William Gibbons and Sons, Wolverhampton

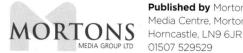

Published by Mortons Media Group Ltd,
Media Centre, Morton Way,
Horncastle, LN9 6JR
01507 529529

Mind, Body & Soul

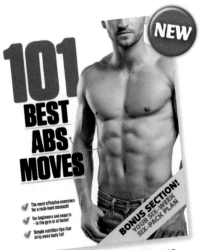

NEW

101 BEST ABS MOVES

- The most effective exercises for a rock-hard stomach!
- For beginners and experts – in the gym or at home!
- Simple nutrition tips that strip away body fat!

BONUS SECTION! YOUR SIX-WEEK SIX-PACK PLAN

When it comes to looking good, few can deny that a washboard six-pack of toned abs looks so much better than a flabby belly. The Complete Guide to Abs explains the simple steps you can take to sculpt your six-pack through a combination of regular exercise and healthy eating. You can also benefit from overall improved health and fitness as part of this straightforward programme.

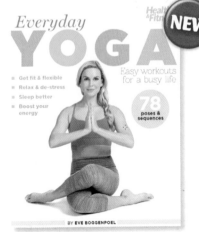

Everyday **YOGA**

Health & Fitness

NEW

Easy workouts for a busy life

- Get fit & flexible
- Relax & de-stress
- Sleep better
- Boost your energy

78 poses & sequences

BY EVE BOGGENPOEL

Until you've experienced it for yourself it's hard to really understand the difference a regular yoga practice can make to your life. People speak of improved flexibility, increased strength, better balance and greater stamina, but the benefits go far beyond the physical. Along with better sleep, deeper relaxation and greater focus you can get a feeling of purpose that is hard to beat.

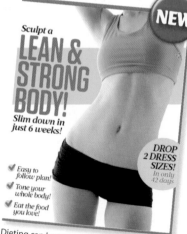

NEW

Sculpt a LEAN & STRONG BODY!

Slim down in just 6 weeks!

- Easy to follow plan!
- Tone your whole body!
- Eat the food you love!

DROP 2 DRESS SIZES! In only 42 days

Dieting can be tough and it's easy to fall off the wagon before you reach your goal - which is why Sculpt a Lean and Strong Body! helps you complete the journey from flabby couch potato to a lean and athletic physique through a simple exercise plan, a generous dietary programme and easily accomplished objectives.

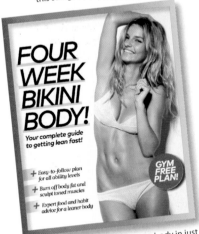

FOUR WEEK BIKINI BODY!

Your complete guide to getting lean fast!

GYM FREE PLAN!

- Easy-to-follow plan for all ability levels
- Burn off body fat and sculpt toned muscles
- Expert food and habit advice for a leaner body

Complete guide to toning up your body in just four weeks. Following a simple step-by-step programme, you'll burn more fat and develop lean, defined muscles. Plus, learn good habits that will make you healthier for life.

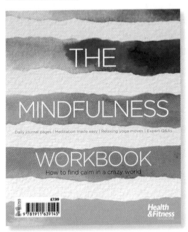

THE MINDFULNESS WORKBOOK

Daily journal pages | Meditation made easy | Relaxing yoga moves | Expert Q&As

How to find calm in a crazy world

£7.99

9 781911 639145

Health & Fitness

If you're not exactly sure what being mindful involves, this is the place to start. Hereyou'll learn the history and main concepts of mindfulness, and get an idea of how your life might look after you learn to live more fully in the moment. Discover the ways mindfulness is used by its many advocates - from celebrities to professors - and learn how it can benefit you too.

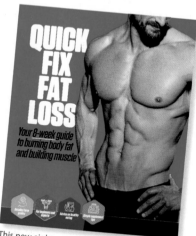

QUICK FIX FAT LOSS

Your 8-week guide to burning body fat and building muscle

This new eight-week training and eating plan that will help you shift body fat fast and allow you to build the body you've always wanted.

Contents

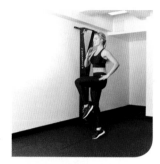

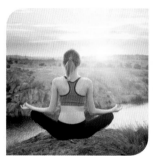

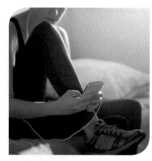

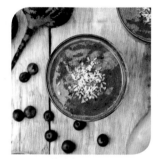

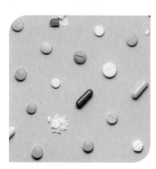

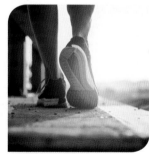

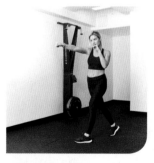

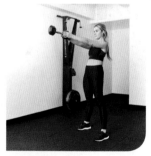

Introduction

Welcome to *7 Laws Of Getting Lean*, your complete guide to stripping away fat fast - and sculpting your best ever body.

Inside this book you will find all the expert insight you need to transform the way you look and feel, including instantly applicable advice on how to make small and sustainable changes to the way you live, sleep, exercise and eat. It'll arm you with all the information you need to get the body you've always wanted.

We've split the book into seven chapters, and each one focuses on an important element of maintaining a lean and healthy physique. This is because if you want to make lasting changes to the way you look and feel, you need to take a holistic approach. You don't have to read the book from cover to cover in one go, but you will find that it is most effective when you apply the ideas in every section to the way you live, eat, rest and exercise.

Good luck, and remember to enjoy the journey!

5 things you need to do before you begin

Clean out your fridge and cupboards to get rid of all those foods and snacks you know you need to avoid in the pursuit of burning body fat quickly. If you're not sure what can stay, we explain the best ways to eat on p32.

Buy a big plastic-free water bottle. Drinking more water is a major factor in priming your body to burn fat. For more information on the amazing power of water in the fight against fat, turn to p36.

Make a playlist of motivational music. Studies have shown exercising to your favourite tunes makes hard training feel easier, and listening to your top tracks can also alleviate stress. Find out more on p24.

If you haven't bought a new pair of running shoes since school then it's time to treat yourself. The right fit will minimise injury risk and allow you to run faster, which is the key to fat loss. Pick the perfect pair with the advice on p63.

The only way to keep pushing yourself in training is to know what you've done before so you can do more next time. Buy a workout diary to record your sessions and track progress. For more motivating tips turn to p14.

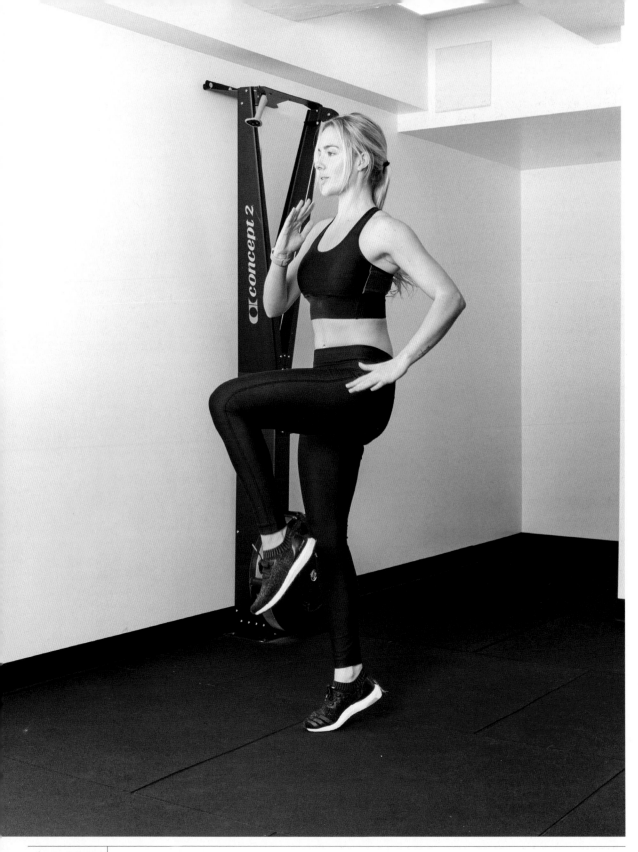

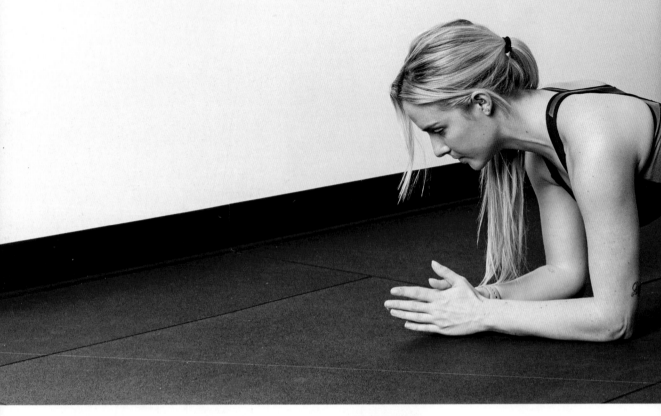

7 fat loss myths you can ignore

'DON'T EAT BREAKFAST'

Skipping breakfast is a big mistake. Breakfast is the most important meal of the day for good reason: your body has been deprived of energy and nutrients for the past eight hours while you've been asleep. Starting your day with good food is crucial, not just for getting into better shape but also for better energy, health, performance and mood. And don't think missing breakfast helps you lose fat – research shows people who do skip it end up consuming more calories over the course of the day.

'YOU NEED TO POUND PAVEMENTS'

The first thing many people do when trying to lose fat is go for long jogs. But while some exercise is better than none, running at a consistent and comfortable speed for an hour or more isn't a very effective way to burn body fat because it doesn't push your body hard enough to use a significant number of calories. And post-session pasta means more calories are consumed than have been burned, which will lead to weight gain, not loss. Turn to p48 to read about the best ways to run.

'WEIGHTS MAKE YOU BULKY'

Weight training is actually one of the very best ways to burn body fat. Why? Lifting weights, especially in high-intensity workouts, gets your heart rate high so you burn calories both during and after your workout, and it also causes the release of hormones that tell your body to release fat for energy and your muscles to get bigger and more defined. Find out more about how weights can help build your new, lean physique – including detailed workouts – on p94.

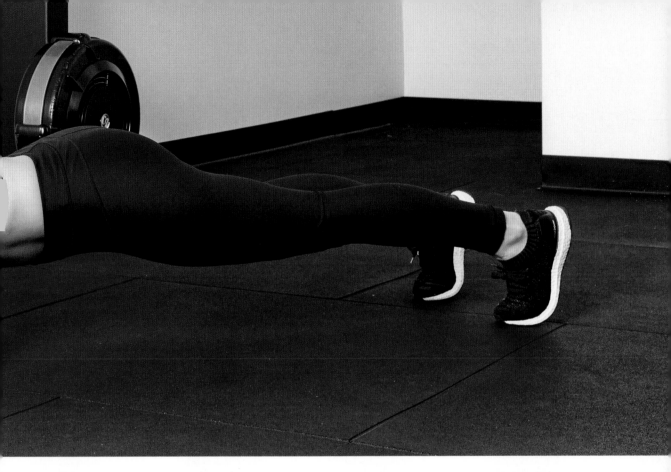

'YOU HAVE TO COUNT CALORIES'

What you eat is important, but the problem with calorie counting is that not all calories are created equal. Without considering where those calories come from – whether carbs, fat or protein – calorie counting is a flawed approach. Still need convincing? What's the better option if you want to lose fat: 250 calories from two boiled eggs and half an avocado (containing quality protein and fat) or 250 calories from a doughnut (almost entirely carbs in the form of sugar)? Find out more on p28.

'YOU MUST AVOID EATING FAT'

Dietary fat was vilified for decades for causing obesity, heart disease and other terminal problems. But the science behind these claims has been discredited and the importance of fats to a healthy and balanced diet is now widely recognised. The one exception is trans fats, which are found in fast food and heavily processed snacks. These are artificially manufactured and not found in nature which means your body doesn't know how to process them and they can cause all kinds of short- and long-term health problems.

'CUT OUT ALL THE CARBS'

With fats back on the menu it was obvious that we'd need a new dietary villain. While cutting down on carbohydrates – especially sugar and heavily processed white bread, rice and pasta – will help you lose fat, cutting out an entire food group permanently is a recipe for disaster. Remember, the best diet is the one you find sustainable and enjoyable. Carbs contain essential vitamins and nutrients, as well as fibre, and can help you perform better in the weights room and on the treadmill.

'YOU NEED FAT LOSS PILLS'

There's a huge market for products that claim to burn body fat without you having to do anything other than pop some pills or drink a special type of tea. If only. Supplements, as their name makes clear, are meant to *supplement* your diet by filling in any nutritional gaps. When you want to get lean, it's exercise and diet – as well as managing stress and getting more sleep – that are by far the most influential factors. But if you're doing everything else right, there are some supplements that can help (p40).

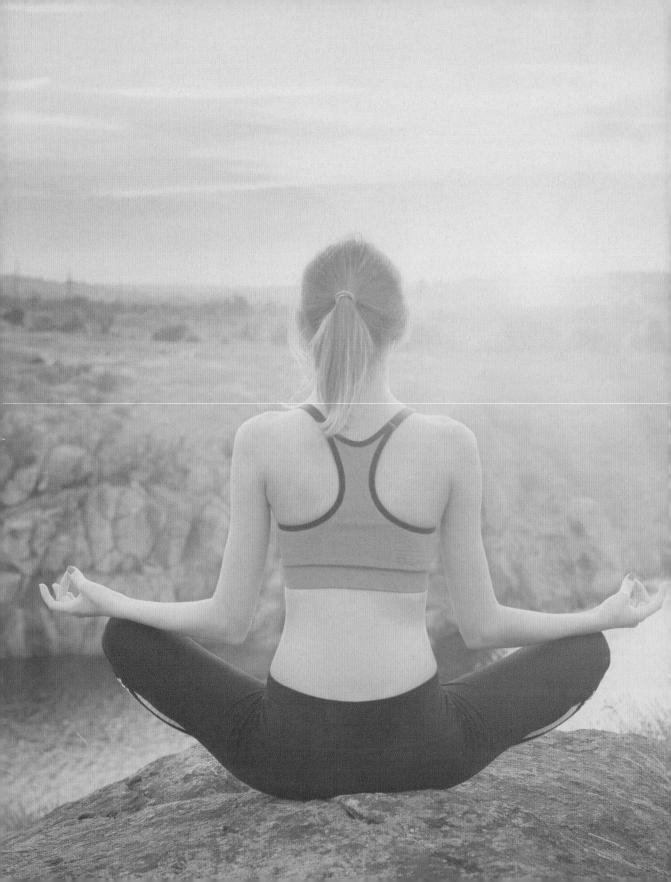

1.

Be kind to your mind

When you want to lose body fat fast, there's something you need to do before anything else (yep, even before you work up a sweat!). That's getting in the right positive mindset, because once you do, every other part of the fat loss puzzle will fall into place. Here's what you need to know to get your head happy and working for you.

When in pursuit of a better body, most people focus primarily on one of two things. They either think about nothing but their muscle tone and whether their arms are looking sufficiently firm and slender, or they fixate on their bottom and belly and whether they're shrinking as quickly as they'd like.

However, in both scenarios, focusing primarily on your physical changes – and how quickly they are occurring – is the wrong approach to take and is likely to lead to disappointment. Whatever your goal, the first thing you need to focus on is your mental outlook and attitude. Because if you start any better-body training and diet plan without the right mentality the wheels will fall off quickly, derailing your best efforts and ensuring you fall short of reaching your fat loss goal.

Undertaking a serious body transformation project is challenging and there will be blips and setbacks along the way. You may even question why you're putting in all this time and effort when the results you want don't appear to be getting any closer! That's why it's absolutely essential to have a positive mentality from the very beginning because it will help you hurdle the obstacles that will inevitably appear in your path.

In this chapter we reveal some helpful tips and insight to enable you to put yourself in the perfect frame of mind to begin your fat loss transformation with the best chance at success, as well as some advice on what you can do to when things go a little awry. Put it into practice and you'll find that no matter what, you can keep moving towards a leaner, more athletic body.

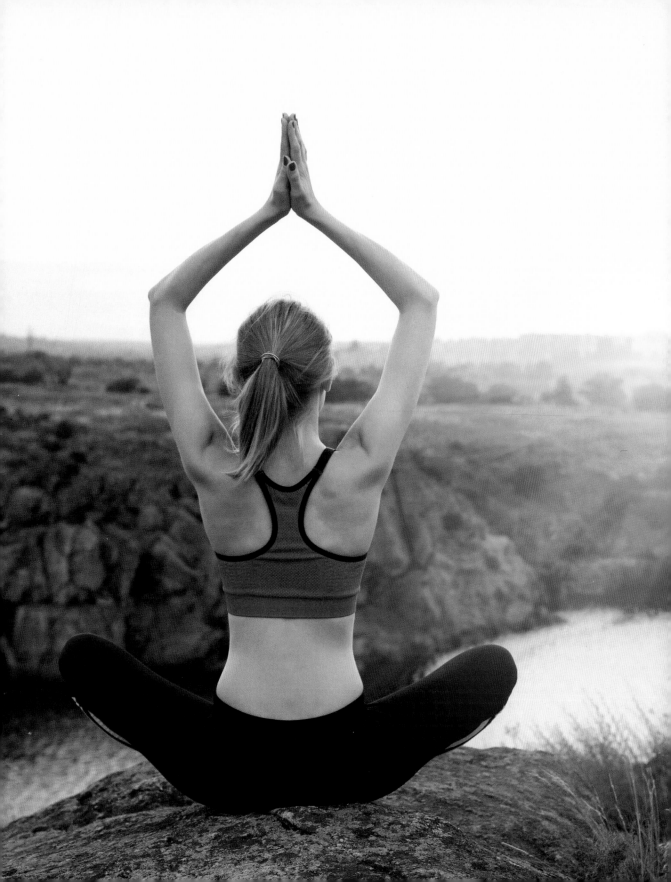

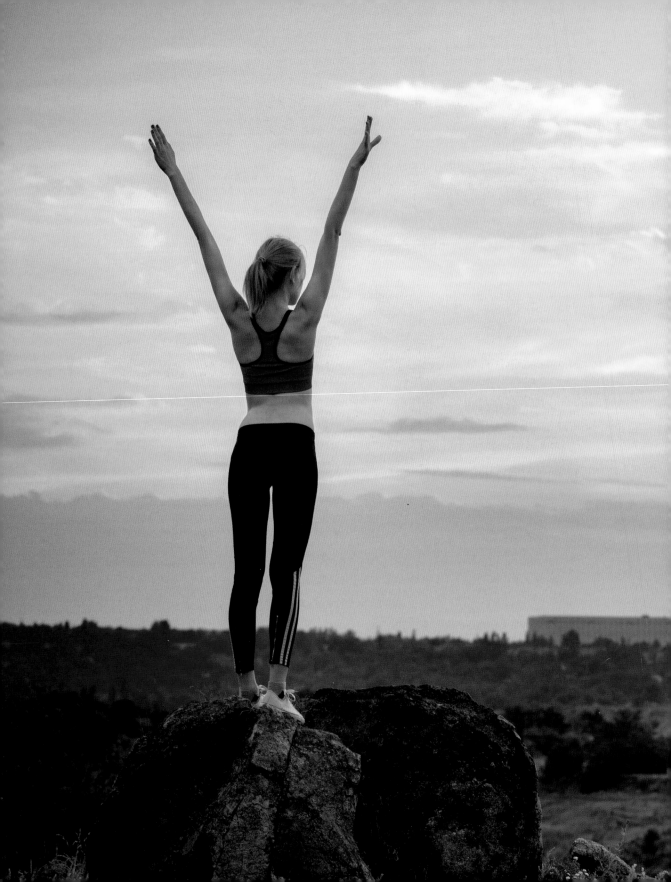

10 ways to stay positive

1

WRITE A FEELGOOD LIST

It's hard to have a positive outlook at the start of your fat loss journey. After all, one of the key reasons you want to lose weight is that you're not happy with the way you look naked. But starting out with a negative mindset won't be productive – instead, write a list of all the things you're grateful for, then jot down all the positive changes you will make to your life by successfully losing weight.

2

SET A REALISTIC GOAL

Once you have your "grateful" list you need to set yourself a challenging yet achievable goal. Not having one means your training will lack focus and your diet plan will be very hard to stick to! This target could be the number of kilos you want to lose, or a certain percentage reduction in body-fat levels – and you also need to have a tough but realistic timeframe in which you plan to achieve it.

3

BREAK IT DOWN INTO STAGES

Your overall goal needs a timeframe. Twelve weeks is enough time to make it happen, but you also need to break this big target down into weekly or fortnightly mini-goals. These milestones will keep your progress moving in the right direction and keep your motivation levels high as you regularly tick off the completion of each one. Work backwards from your big goal to come up with mini-ones.

4

ENLIST SOME SUPPORT

A great way to get - and stay - motivated is to enlist the support of friends and family. Tell your close circle about your fat loss goal and why you are undertaking it to get them onside to support you. If they know what and why you're doing it will help in many ways, especially when you are finding it hard to keep going, and will also make them less likely to twist your arm to do things that will be detrimental to your chances of success.

5

GET A FRIEND INVOLVED

Even better than getting support from your friends is signing up one or more of them to get into better shape with you. Numerous studies have reported that working out with someone else increases the motivation to exercise in the first place, and that you also work out harder and more efficiently than when you do it alone. A little bit of friendly support can be the extra spur you need to train harder and eat better to strip away fat.

6 BOOK IN YOUR GYM SESSIONS

Every Sunday spend 10 minutes booking the week's workout sessions into your work diary. Having them down in black and white and giving them the same importance as your social and professional commitments means you will treat them as such and never have the excuse to skip a session. The most important element when trying to change your body for the better is consistency, and the more consistent you can be with your exercise, the faster you'll burn fat.

7 KEEP A TRAINING DIARY

Logging your progress is a fantastic way to stay on top of your fat loss challenge. After each training session, write down the reps you completed for each exercise, or the distance and time of your cardio workout. You can also record other data such as energy levels, motivation levels, hours of sleep and other important lifestyle factors to have a detailed record of how you feel as well as how you look. You'll know at a glance if you're improving, and get an idea of what to change if not.

8 TAKE PROGRESS PHOTOS

Another great way to track your progress and stay motivated is to take weekly progress shots of your body. Seeing how your body changes for the better week by week can be incredibly inspiring and keep you focused on moving closer to your goal. Just make sure you take the photo on the same day each week at the same time, ideally in the same place and with the same lighting. This will give you the most accurate image of how you're doing.

9 REWARD YOUR EFFORTS

If you have previously struggled with motivation levels, there are some simple tricks you can use to make this attempt more successful. One could be to put aside a fiver every time you complete a workout. It might not seem much, but the simple act of doing so gives you a reason to train, and the cash will soon add up. Four sessions a week for 12 weeks gives you £240, which will go some way towards the new wardrobe you're going to need.

10 LEARN TO LOVE THE PROCESS

Spending months working towards a leaner body is not easy - in fact it can be extremely hard at times, which is why so many people start to hate the process and even give up. Doing a bit more exercise and keeping a closer eye on what you eat isn't the short-term solution; it should be the starting point of positive lifestyle changes that will make you fitter, healthier and happier for good. Do the type of training you enjoy and if you find yourself resenting the gym, find a better way to work out.

GET BACK ON YOUR FEET FAST

At some point during your fat loss challenge it's almost inevitable that something will happen that threatens to ruin your efforts. It might be an unplanned night out of too much wine or a takeaway after a hard day. That, in isolation, isn't a huge problem – but only if you get back on your programme the very next day. A cheat meal won't trash your chances of shedding fat fast, but if it turns into a cheat day or even a cheat week, you will be undoing your hard work up to that point. Consistency is crucial, so if you eat well and exercise hard most of the time, an occasional setback won't be too much of a problem... just don't make it a habit.

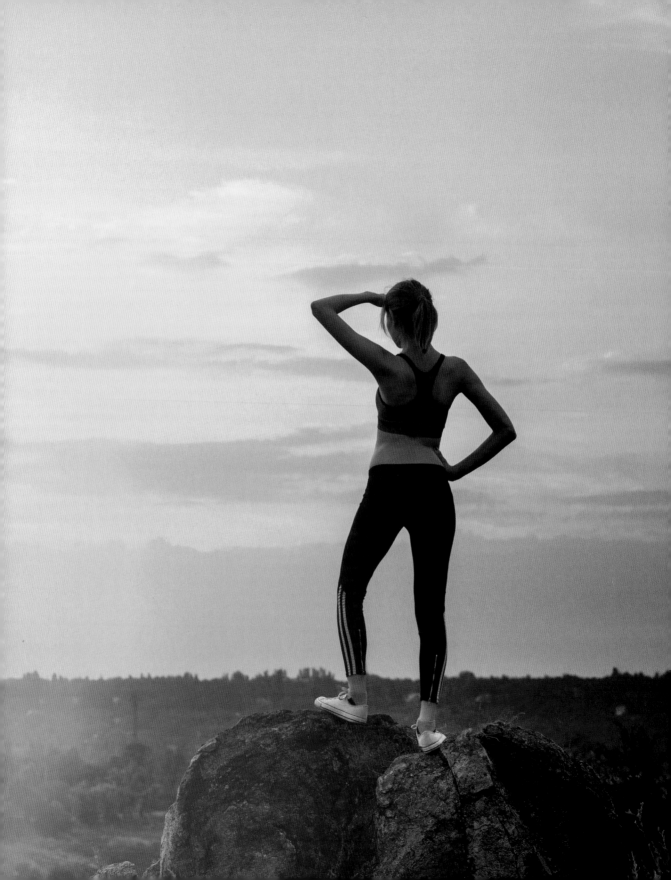

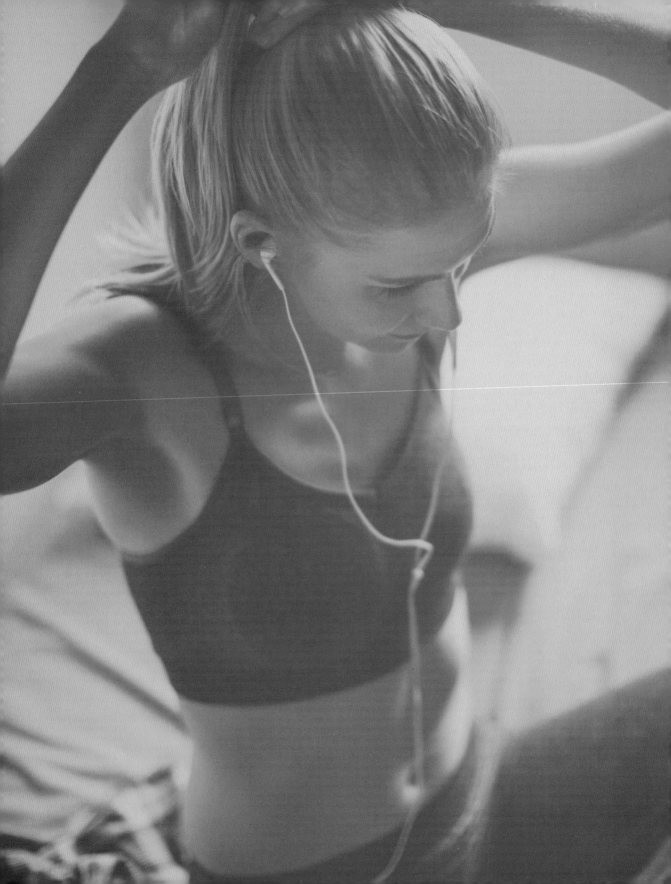

2.
Manage your lifestyle

Even if you exercise for an hour daily there's still another 23 hours in the day, and it's your actions during this 96% of your time that determines how successful your fat loss journey will be. Luckily, by making some small lifestyle changes you can make a big impact on how much body fat you burn – and how quickly. Read on to find out more.

The unfortunate truth for anyone looking to get leaner is that your body doesn't want to be lean, and it will fight hard to maintain relatively high body-fat levels. That's good news from an evolutionary point of view – it's this ability to store energy as fat that enabled our ancestors to survive long periods of famine – but it's bad news if you want to slim down! While it can be hard to shift body fat, though (especially from those body areas like the bottom and thighs, which for many people is where fat sticks around most stubbornly) it's by no means impossible.

In later chapters you will discover the best exercise approaches to shift body fat fast, which means high-intensity cardio sessions and circuit-based resistance workouts. You'll also find a smart and sustainable approach to eating that gives your body all the essential nutrients it needs for you to perform at your best, both physically and mentally, while also freeing up body fat to be used for fuel.

However, before you start your new workout plan or clean out to your cupboards to make space for all the healthy food you will need, it's vital that you make some small but significant changes to your lifestyle to give yourself the best chance of getting lean quickly. Changing your lifestyle might sound like a bit of an ordeal, but in reality the required changes are quick and easy and will still have a profound and positive impact on every area of your life. If you follow our advice on how to recover faster from exercise, how to minimise your daily exposure to stress and better manage it when it happens, and how to sleep better for longer so you wake up every morning not only feeling fully energised, it'll help you feel stronger, healthier and more motivated.

These simple changes will make it much easier for you to strip away body fat and build a leaner, more toned body quickly. That's because to lose fat fast you need every aspect of your life to be working towards this goal. Recover quicker and you'll be motivated to start the next session when it comes around. Keep your stress levels down and you'll lower your levels of the stress hormone cortisol, a high level of which encourages your body to hold on to fat stores and even to add to them. And sleeping deeper for longer every night will give you more energy to exercise and more motivation to stick to the best nutrition plan to change your body for the better.

Turn the page and follow our advice to live a fitter, healthier and happier life.

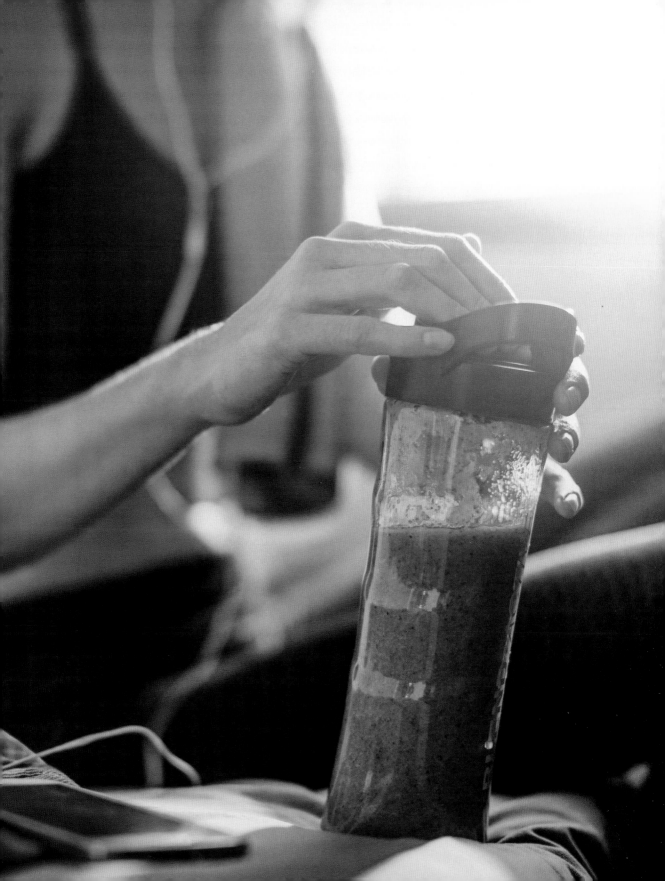

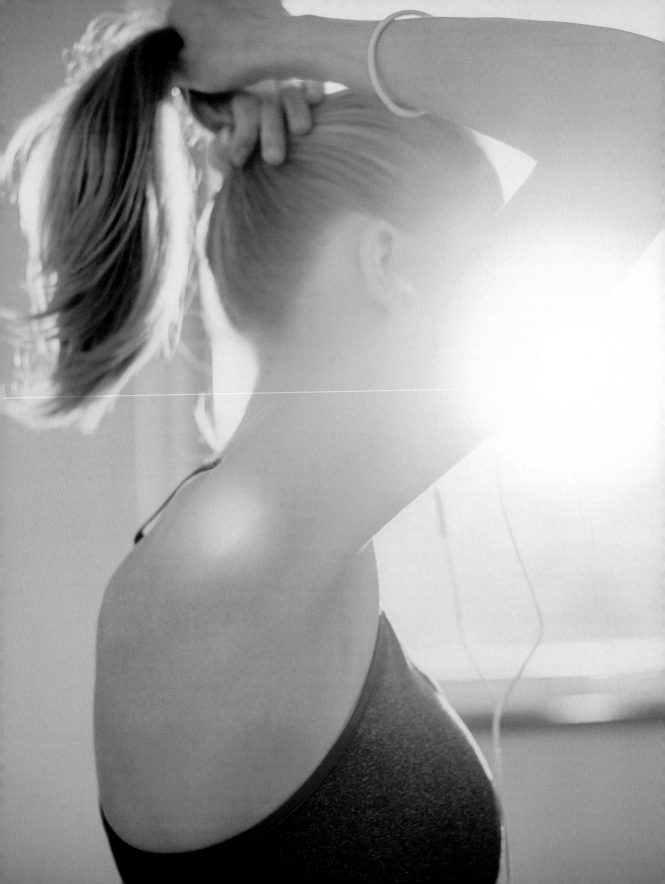

Be kind to your body

Working out takes a lot out of you, both physically and mentally. But for the best fat loss results you need to exercise consistently, so try these five recovery strategies so you're ready to give every session all you've got

WARM UP AND DOWN

Jumping straight into a workout, especially a high-intensity cardio or circuit session, without warming up means it's only a matter of time until you get injured. And good luck trying to get lean when you're laid up in bed! Warming up before exercise, and warming down afterwards, helps your body move from a resting state to an active one and back again, and is an important part of the preparation and recovery process. Do it properly and you won't regret it.

BE SMART WITH STRETCHES

Later in this book we'll explain why you shouldn't do static stretches before exercise, but instead favour dynamic ones that better mimic movement patterns you'll follow during the main workout. But that doesn't mean that static stretching doesn't have a part to play in speeding up your recovery. For example, the day after a hard session try doing some light activity, such as a jog, then some static stretching to ease your muscles.

DRINK MORE WATER

To sculpt a better body you need to drink more water every day. Aim for at least two litres on non-training days, and three litres or more on training days. Drinking more water keeps your body hydrated, which will aid your mood and concentration levels (making that hard session more enjoyable) and help you get leaner. Carry a big bottle around with you all day, sipping from it frequently. And don't be afraid to refill it multiple times every day.

WORK ON YOUR MOBILITY

Poor joint mobility, especially in your shoulders, hips and ankles, can have a serious negative impact on the efficiency of your exercise – which is a key to faster fat loss – as well as increasing your risk of pain and injury. Make mobility work a big part of your post-session warm-down, or do some on rest days as part of your "active recovery" strategy. A good foam roller isn't too expensive and can be worth its weight in gold if it keeps you injury- and pain-free.

TAKE A DEEP BATH

Many athletes around the world swear that having an ice bath after a match, competition or hard training session helps them recover faster. Science doesn't fully support this anecdotal evidence, but there's no harm in you alternating between hot and cold water during your post-session shower to see if it works for you. Or at the end of the day, run a deep hot bath with Epsom salts to help revive sore and aching muscles.

Say goodbye to stress

Modern life is more stressful than ever, with working days growing longer as you try to juggle your personal and professional life. But high stress levels will undermine your fat loss efforts, so try these five tips to reduce some of more avoidable causes of stress

WORK UP A QUICK SWEAT

Sometimes you might feel far too busy and stressed to just drop everything at work or at home so you can go and exercise. But doing so will help not only make you slimmer, it will also give your brain some much-needed downtime. Even just a short but intense 20-minute workout can be enough to give you a more positive outlook, and help you get some perspective so you'll manage your time better to keep stress at arm's length.

FOCUS ON ONE JOB AT A TIME

When your in-tray begins to spill over it often leads to working longer hours...as well as snacking and eating convenience foods or takeaways at your desk! Too many late nights too often will seriously hamper your efforts to build a leaner body. So instead, prioritise your most important tasks of the day and get them ticked off your to-do list. The non-urgent stuff can either be delegated or done when things settle down.

MAKE MORE TIME FOR YOU

Today many of us struggle to have half as much downtime as we'd like – and most of us would like to improve our work-life balance. But to live a more stress-free life, or at least be better able to deal with stress when it inevitably arises, requires you to find time to do more of the things you love and make you happy. It doesn't matter what that hobby, activity or pursuit is, so long as it's a passion of yours. Schedule in some "me time" and your stress levels will plummet.

TURN THE MUSIC UP LOUD

Sometimes you might only have five minutes of spare time to yourself between meetings and picking up the kids or planning an event. Use that precious time to perfection by putting on your favourite upbeat song, turning up the volume and closing your eyes. Numerous studies have shown a direct and positive correlation between listening music and elevated mood and decreased anxiety. Even better, create a whole playlist of feelgood tunes.

GO TO BED A LITTLE EARLIER

Most people think there are two things that affect how quickly you lose weight: exercise and diet. If asked to name a third factor they might say supplements. But when you want to strip away body fat (or build muscle for that matter) it's getting enough sleep every night that's crucial. Insufficient or poor-quality sleep increases stress levels, your risk of obesity and many other health problems. Turn the page to find out how you can start to sleep better.

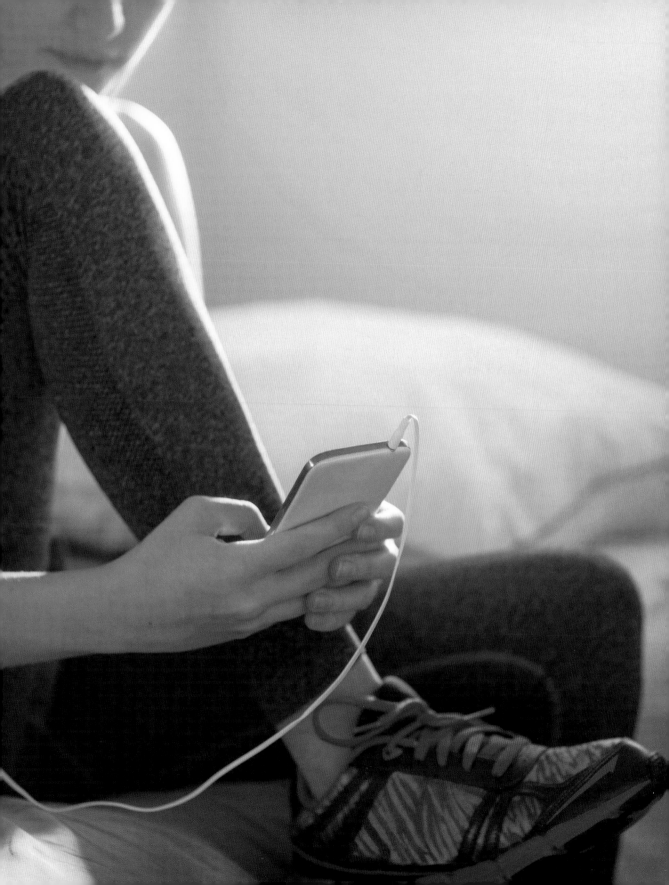

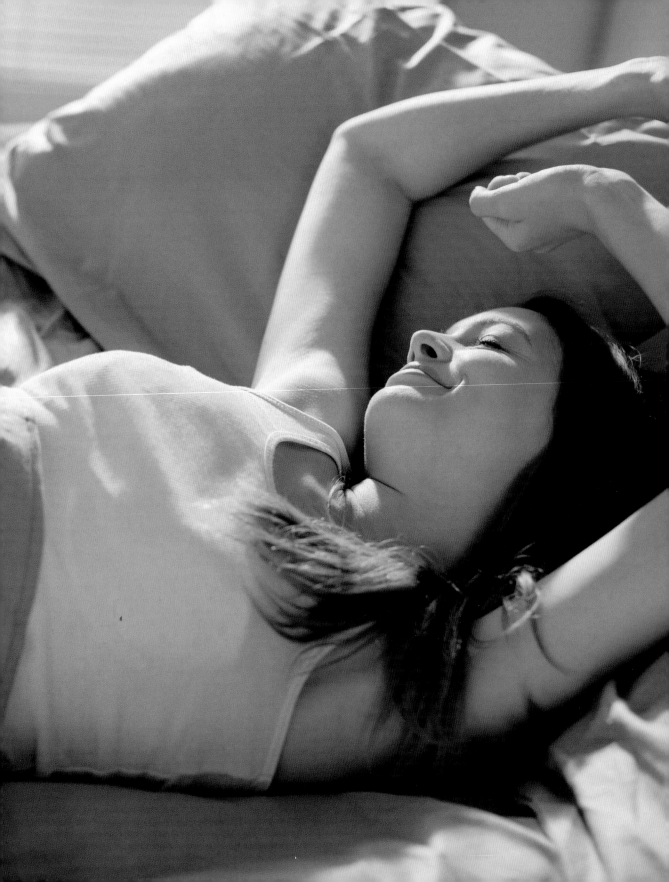

Sleep tight every night

Getting quality sleep every night will give you the energy and motivation to do what it takes to reduce body fat. Use these better-sleep tips from Shawn Stevenson, author of *Sleep Smarter: 21 Essential Strategies To Sleep Your Way To A Better Body, Better Health And Bigger Success*

SWITCH OFF THE SCREENS

Cutting back on screen use before bed is the best thing you can do to improve sleep quantity and quality. Laptops and monitors emit artificial blue light that triggers your body to produce more daytime hormones, such as cortisol, and produce less melatonin, the hormone that induces sleep. In a study, subjects who read a book on a tablet took longer to fall asleep and had less REM (the deep, restorative stage) sleep than those who read a paper book.

CUT BACK ON THE BOOZE

As well as the empty calories alcohol brings, it has a significant impact on sleep quality. Drinking booze close to bedtime causes you to stay below normal levels of REM sleep during the first stage of sleep, and then there's an "REM rebound" that puts sleep *above* normal REM as your body tries to sort things out. It's why you can sleep for hours after a few glasses of wine but still wake up exhausted.

WORK OUT BEFORE WORK

If you want to sleep better at night, try working out first thing in the morning. One big issue with working out in the evening is that it raises your core body temperature, and it can take four to six hours for it to come down again. Your body has a regulation process that lowers your core temperature to create the optimal conditions for sleep, and raising it too close to bedtime can mess up that process and prevent you getting the best sleep possible.

AVOID CARBS BEFORE BED

You will find out more about carbs and the role they play in fat loss in the Nutrition chapter (p28) but for now, know that a big serving of carbs right before bed is one of the main ways to negatively affect sleep. It will cause a big blood sugar spike once you have fallen asleep, which is then likely to pull you out of the deeper, restorative stages of sleep and make it difficult to drift back into them.

GET MORE PHYSICAL

Sex induces sleep because an orgasm releases a cascade of feelgood chemicals, which have a calming effect that counters the stimulating effects of the stress hormone cortisol, as well as prolactin, a hormone linked to sexual satisfaction and better sleep. Want more sex? Turn off the box: a study of 500 Italian couples found those without a TV in the bedroom have twice as much sex as couples who do.

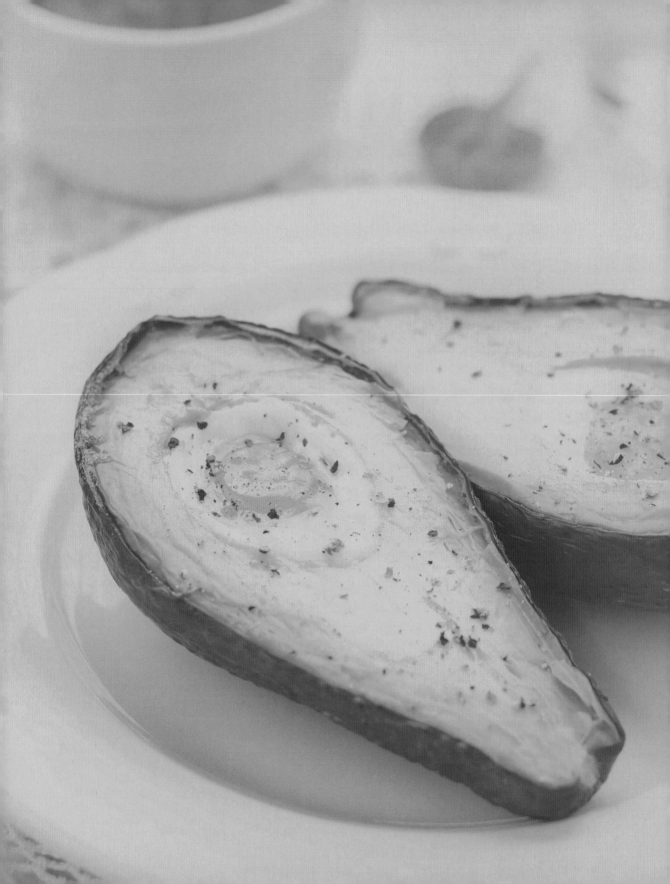

3.
Fight fat with food

The key to reducing body fat through your diet is to eat a wide variety of fresh food and create a long-term plan that's sustainable and enjoyable. The truth is that you can't fight fat with a fad diet, but if you make a few simple adjustments to the way you eat, you'll see your waistline shrink – without giving up all the foods you love!

Here's the reality: it doesn't matter how hard you train in the gym if you don't put the same time, effort and focus into what you do in the kitchen. The old saying that "you can't out-train a bad diet" is something of a cliché, but like most clichés it's rooted in truth. And if you want to make big changes to how you look – and as quickly as possible – then you need to start thinking more about mealtimes.

The problem is that what to eat and when can seem a complicated business. But don't worry: eating for a better body really isn't as confusing as some people make out. Everything you need to know is explained in this chapter, so you'll have all the information you need to put in place some better eating strategies to strip away body fat at a steady and sustainable rate.

This chapter starts with the seven nutrition principles you need to follow to start eating for a leaner body .After that we've put together a guide to some easy, healthy daily habits you can adopt so that eating well at each and every meal becomes second nature.

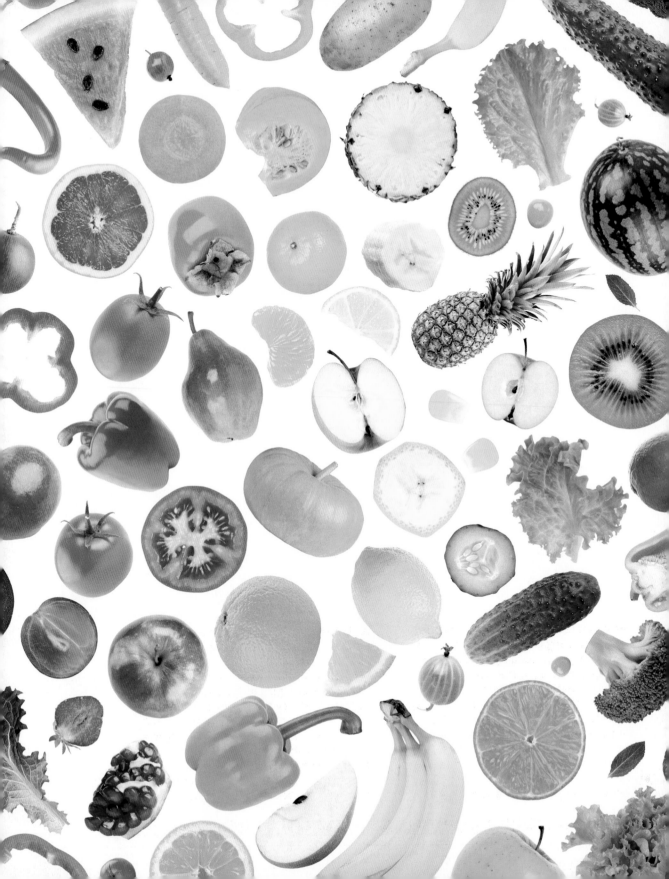

7 rules of eating for fat loss

Follow these seven fat-burning food strategies to transform your body

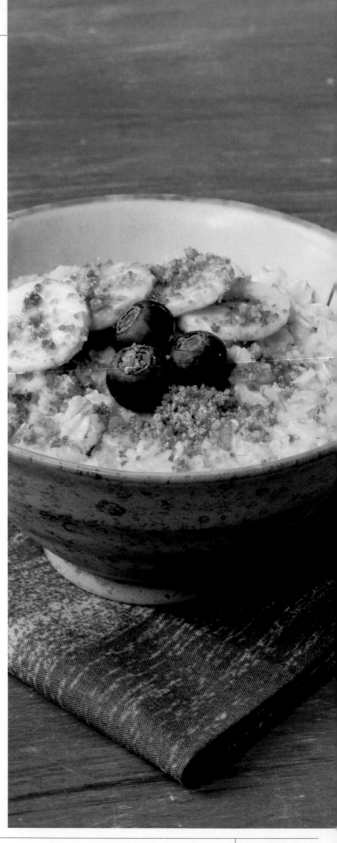

NEVER SKIP BREAKFAST

As we saw in the fat loss myths on p8, there's a reason breakfast is known as the most important meal of the day. It might seem to make sense to skip it when trying to lose fat – hey, that's a big wodge of calories you're not getting, right? – but both scientists and people who've tried that know it doesn't work: research shows that people who don't eat brekkie consume more calories over the course of the entire day than those who do.

Breakfast kick-starts your body's processes, including fat-burning metabolism, after all those hours spent asleep, helping your body burn fat throughout the day. It will also keep blood sugar levels steady so you aren't tempted to eat high-sugar and high-fat foods. Eating a good breakfast also improves your focus, motivation and willpower, and you need all three to ensure you stick to your exercise and healthy eating plans.

KEEP IT NATURAL

All the food you buy from now on should be in its natural form, or as close to it as possible. That means stocking your fridge with lean red and white meat, fish, eggs and as many varieties and colours of veg as you can get your hands on. You'll know from experience that going to

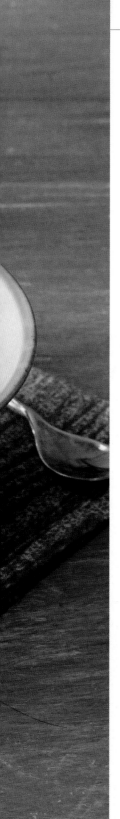

the supermarket when hungry always results in your trolley getting loaded with foods and snacks that are high in sugar and calories but low in the essential nutrients your body needs to get and stay lean. So only ever shop when you've recently eaten, or do a big online shop once a week so you only buy the healthier foods you know you need.

Eating a diet based entirely around natural whole foods, and avoiding all high-carb, high-fat convenience foods, will ensure your body gets the maximum amount of nutrients but not the excess calories so you can start to shift those excess kilos.

DON'T FOCUS ON CALORIES

For years the concept that to lose weight you should count calories prevailed. But once you realise that not all calories are created equal, you see the flaw in this system. A litre tub of ice cream has about 2,000 calories, but if you get your daily calorie intake by splitting that over three meals, that's not as good for fat loss – or your overall health! – as getting the same amount of calories from lean meat and fish, fresh vegetables and wholegrain carbs.

That's an extreme example, of course, but the face remains that your body needs lots of high-quality protein and fats (which are calorie-dense) to support your exercise efforts and aid recovery so you can keep moving towards your goal. If you're unsure how this works in practice, just follow the next four rules – you won't go far wrong.

EAT MORE PROTEIN

Remember, the best and fastest way to change your body shape is to exercise several times a week and support your efforts with a healthy balanced diet, and protein is a big part of that. If you don't eat enough good-quality protein – think red and white meat, fish and eggs – then you're unlikely to make the progress you want as quickly as you'd like.

Aim for a fist-sized serving of protein for every meal, and spend a little more money if you can to buy organic and grass-fed produce because it contains more vitamins, minerals and omega 3 fatty acids, which will also help you burn fat. And don't worry - although protein does help build muscle, eating more of it won't make you bulky. In fact, it's likely to have the

opposite effect, because when you eat protein you feel fuller for longer, which will help you manage the quantity of food that you consume.

EAT MORE VEG

No messing around here: veg is fantastic. If you struggle to get your five-a-day then up your game, because you need to have veg – and a wide variety of it – with every meal you eat. It's packed with the vitamins and minerals your body demands after training, as well as fibre to keep you feeling fuller for longer and stabilise your blood sugar levels so you won't be tempted by sweet snacks.

If you dislike vegetables there are simple ways to make them more palatable. Try adding butter on the plate to improve flavour and help vitamin absorption, or cook them with garlic, chilli or any herbs and spices to add some flavour.

FAT IS YOUR FRIEND

The idea that eating fat made you fat took hold in the 1970s and has proved hard to shift. But as we explained in the fat loss myths on p9, we now know now that it isn't true (and we've been left with a legacy of "low-fat" foods that won't help you lose weight). Fats are an important part of a healthy diet – especially with regards to better hormone function, which enables you to burn body fat more efficiently. You can get them from a variety of sources, including dairy, meat, natural oils and avocado – but you do still need to avoid man-made trans fats (the kind used in heavily processed food such as biscuits). These fats won't help fuel your workouts or weight loss and are associated with higher risks of health problems like heart disease, strokes and diabetes.

STOP DRINKING SUGAR

One easy way to boost your chances of getting lean is to stop drinking so many calories, especially those found in fizzy drinks and processed fruit juices. These drinks have little to no nutritional value and should be completely avoided if you care about being lean – and about your overall health for that matter. Ideally, you should drink only three things: water (aim for at least two litres per day, and even more on days you work out); coffee (black is best); and tea (green is great, four sugars is bad).

Build healthy habits

Implement these new lifestyle routines to stack your odds in favour of sculpting a lean and toned physique

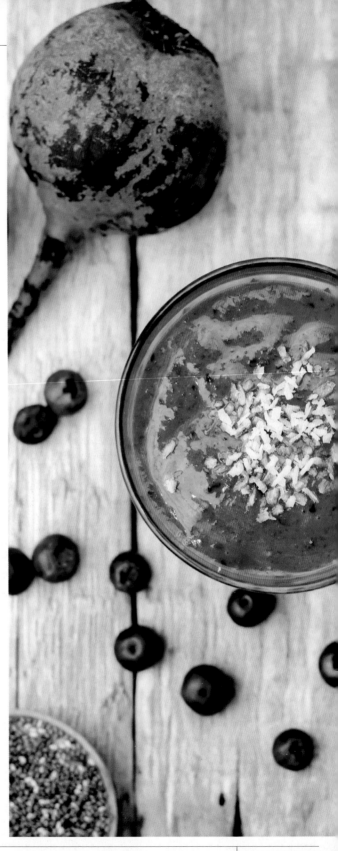

WAKE UP WITH WATER

As soon as you get up – even before you go to the loo – down a pint of cold water. You wake in a dehydrated state and it's crucial to replace the water you've lost overnight (through sweating and simply breathing) as quickly as you can. Dehydration is a leading cause of poor mental and physical performance, both of which you want to avoid to stay focused and motivated for your fat loss journey. Always carry a big bottle of water around with you and sip from it constantly throughout the day to keep hydrated at all times.

EAT AT THE SAME TIMES

You don't need to time your meals like clockwork but try to eat breakfast, lunch and dinner at roughly the same times each day. This will soon establish a regular routine where you think nothing of taking the time to sit down and eat properly. Doing this can go a long way towards maximising the nutritional impact of the wholesome food you're consuming, whereas eating in a rushed or stressed state won't.

Eating at set times also removes the risk that you'll skip meals or go for long periods without eating anything, which more often than not results in cravings for high-sugar and high-fat snacks and convenience foods.

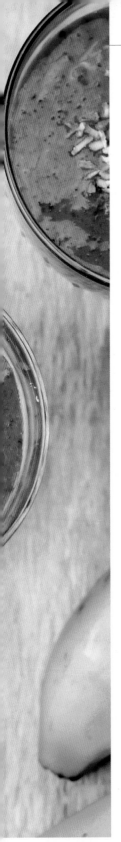

KEEP A FOOD DIARY

If you are really struggling to stay on top of your diet, start writing a food diary. You don't need to write down every single calorie you consume, or even the number of grams of protein you've eaten. A simple ballpark figure of what you ate and how much of it, as well as notes on how you feel – especially your energy and motivation levels – will give you a good steer on where you are going right or what you might be doing wrong, allowing you to make small and sensible changes to your nutritional approach and keep moving closer to finding the best dietary strategy for you.

DOUBLE DOWN AT DINNER

When making dinner, double the ingredients and make two portions so that you will have leftovers ready for tomorrow's lunch. This will not only save you time and money, it will also make it much easier for you to eat healthily and keep you on the path to significant fat loss. An even better strategy, if you have time, is to batch-cook two or three different meals at the weekend and keep them in the fridge or freezer, then simply reheat them throughout the week.

BE CLEVER WITH CARBS

We're certainly not going to tell you to eliminate all carbohydrates from your diet for the rest of your life. That would be mean – carbs are delicious, after all – and, as we said earlier (fat loss myths, p9) it isn't even necessary.

Remember, a fat loss diet is only effective if you stick to it, and limiting yourself to only ever eating salmon and broccoli will see the wheels come off within 48 hours, at most. That said, you do need to be smart when selecting the carbs you eat. It's best to avoid most types of sugar, and limit consumption of fast-release carbs, like processed white bread, pasta and rice, all of which have been stripped of many of their nutrients and much of their fibre content. This means the energy from these carbs enters your bloodstream quicker and causes a blood sugar spike.

To lose fat faster you want blood sugar levels that are as stable as possible. So your carbs should come from slow-release sources, like sweet potatoes and brown rice, as well as plenty of fibre-rich, nutrient-dense veg.

Basically, you can't eat too many vegetables when following this plan. The more the better.

EATING OUT MADE EASY

It's almost inevitable that while you're following a lean-body plan like this one, you'll be invited out for a dinner that you can't (and don't want to) turn down. But this needn't be a cause of stress or fear that you'll be jeopardising your fat loss efforts. Most restaurants will serve you whatever you want, so long as it's on the menu somewhere (and you ask nicely). So never be afraid to ask to swap a side of fries for a mixed salad, a creamy sauce for a spicy one, or even for an extra big serving of grilled veg to go with your chicken or fish. Ordering the healthiest option possible will keep you progressing without you feeling any concern or guilt about undoing your hard work in the gym. So sit back, relax, and enjoy your meal even more because you haven't had to cook it (and don't have to do the washing-up).

GO EASY ON BOOZE

The chances are you will also be invited out by a friend for drinks at some point – a birthday, a promotion, it's Friday – but it's vital to ensure all your hard work isn't wasted by a night on the town. To reach your goals fast it's best not to drink alcohol at all, at least not until you're getting close to having the body you want.

However, if the occasion or situation warrants you raising a glass, then stick to a clear spirit and a low-calorie mixer. Vodka and soda or gin and tonic are your best bet – always ask for a big wedge of lime, because it will slightly blunt the sugar spike from the booze – or a small glass of red wine. Beer, cider and sugary cocktails are best avoided.

Many people find it almost impossible to have just a single drink and stop, and the more you drink the more calories you pour down your neck that will ultimately end up on your bottom and thighs. More than that, you're more likely to make poor food choices under the influence as your blood sugar levels crash and hunger strikes. Are you really going to make the gym tomorrow with a raging hangover? Have one drink, if you must, then switch to water or go home to avoid further temptation. For more about booze and its effects turn to p38.

Fight fat with water

If you want to lose fat faster then you need to avoid dehydration – here's why and how

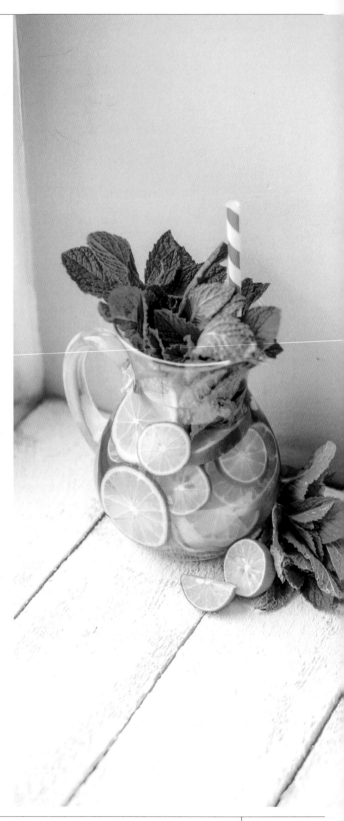

When you're trying hard to slim down, you need as many factors to be in your favour as possible. And for your body to efficiently and effectively tap into fat stores to use of fuel it needs to be performing at its best, which means it needs to be hydrated. Indeed, being dehydrated can seriously damage your fat loss efforts because your body will be desperately trying to fix this problem, so burning fat drops down its priority list. What's more, dehydration affects both physical and mental performance, so you'll struggle with motivation and focus to train and eat well. And that's bad news for your body! Here's what you need to know.

WHY DOES MY BODY NEED WATER?

The human body is approximately 60% water, so you're more water than anything else. While you can go weeks without food, you won't survive more than a few days without water. The reasons include its role in protecting and cushioning the brain, spinal column and other tissues, regulating body temperature, lubricating joints, and removing toxins and waste products through perspiration and excretion, among many others. Most water leaves your body through perspiration and excretion (sweat and urine), but significant quantities are also lost through breathing as water vapour. Adequate water intake is required daily to prevent dehydration, which can lead to a rapid decline in mental and physical performance. It's very easy to lose a lot of body water when training at high intensity, especially in hot conditions.

HOW MUCH WATER DO I NEED EACH DAY?
The National Health Service in Britain recommends drinking eight medium-sized glasses of water a day, but this is obviously only a generic guide and how much you need exactly will depend on body size, activity level, temperature, humidity, diet and myriad other factors.

Most of your daily fluid intake doesn't actually come from drinking plain water but instead from the food you eat and other beverages. For example, a medium banana contains 90ml of water, as does 100g of tomatoes. The United States National Research Council's recommended total daily water intake – which is 3.7 litres for men and 2.7 litres for women – includes water from food and all other sources.

And drinking more water can help you lose weight: numerous studies have shown that drinking 500ml of water at mealtimes is conducive to weight loss, possibly because it makes you feel full sooner so you don't overeat.

WHAT HAPPENS WHEN I GET DEHYDRATED?
The less water in your body, the thicker your blood. This forces your heart to pump harder to deliver oxygen to your brain, organs, muscles and every cell in your body. If you're dehydrated your body will be going haywire trying to fix the problem and as dehydration gets worse you'll feel thirsty, dizzy and irritable and have a headache. Without water at this point your condition will worsen into fatigue and exhaustion, with poor motor function so you'll be clumsy and uncoordinated. None of this will help you exercise, cook healthy meals or do anything else!

HOW DOES DEHYDRATION AFFECT HOW I PERFORM?
Even a 1% decline in fluids as a percentage of total bodyweight can negatively impair performance, according to research from the California University of Pennsylvania, while a decline of 3% or higher significantly increases the risk of heat exhaustion or heat stroke.

Dehydration of 2% impairs mental performance in tasks that require attention, psychomotor and immediate memory skills, according to a study published in the *American Journal Of The College Of Nutrition*, which is no surprise because your brain is predominantly water. The more activity you do and the higher the temperature, the more your daily fluid intake must increase to avoid dehydration.

Research in the journal *Nutrition* advises drinking 200ml to 285ml of water for every ten to 20 minutes of moderate exercise. If it's hot and you're working out at a high intensity then you will need more, and you may need electrolytes too (see below).

HOW DO I KNOW IF I AM DEHYDRATED?
The first and most obvious sign is that you feel thirsty. At the onset of thirst you should drink water, whether you're at work, the gym or outdoors. During intense exercise, or when training in hot and humid conditions, it can be very difficult to consume as much water as you are losing through sweating and breathing. This is why it's so important to start any activity in a fully hydrated state, and prioritise replacing lost fluids as soon as you're finished.

The colour of your urine is also a good indicator of hydration levels: a light yellow colour means you're adequately hydrated, and the darker the colour the more water you need. If it's any other colour, by the way, you should call your doctor.

WHY MIGHT I NEED ELECTROLYTES?
When we sweat we lose important minerals such as sodium and potassium, which are found in your blood and – among other things – regulate body water levels. If you're training for less than an hour in average temperature and humidity you'll be fine to rehydrate with water, but when training is longer, more intense or in hotter conditions, taking on around 1.7g to 2.9g of electrolytes per litre of water helps your body absorb fluids more quickly, according to research in the journal *Sports Medicine*. Another study, published in the *Journal Of The International Society Of Sports Nutrition*, found that pure coconut water and coconut drinks made from concentrate were as effective as sugar-based sports drinks at aiding rehydration.

Booze and your body

If you're serious about sculpting a fitter, healthier and leaner body, science says you should think twice about that glass of wine – especially after exercise

After a long, hard day and a tough workout nothing quite quenches your thirst like a well-made cocktail. You know that water, an electrolyte drink or a protein shake would be better for you, but sometimes only a "real" drink can hit the spot. Indeed, there is a direct correlation between people who work out more and alcohol consumption, says research published in the *American Journal Of Health Promotion*. But how detrimental to your training, and your fitness goals, is a post-exercise social drink? We're afraid we have some bad news.

INCREASED FAT STORAGE

Drinking too much too often will end your ambitions of getting lean because it will make you fatter. A gram of alcohol contains seven calories, just two less than a gram of fat, but unlike fats – which contain vitamins and other compounds essential to good health – alcohol calories contain nothing else of nutritional value, just lots of energy you don't need. With around 180 calories per 250ml glass of wine and 200 calories in a pint of beer, these excess calories cause weight gain and obesity, according to the journal *Clinical Laboratory Sciences*.

DELAYED RECOVERY

Anyone who has ever had a few too many will know that even simple tasks the morning after, like getting out of bed, require superhuman efforts. So drinking after a tough workout will derail the next day's exercise efforts – but the effects can last well into the day after that too. The negative impact is even more pronounced if you are training in an endurance discipline, according to research published in the journal *Sports Medicine*, because alcohol slows the speed at which your body recovers. This affects muscle recovery but also further compromises your immune system, which is already weakened by your endurance efforts, making it harder for you to fight off illness.

BAD FOOD CRAVINGS

After training, your blood sugar levels are low because a lot of your readily available energy stores are emptied. A night of drinking lowers them further, so you wake the next morning in a state of hypoglycaemia (very low blood sugar levels), according to the journal *Diabetes Care*. This is one reason we crave sugary and fatty foods when hungover. Indulging that urge will spike and then crash blood sugar levels, so you'll struggle to motivate yourself to exercise – and even if you do, lower energy levels will produce poor performance. Have a high-protein breakfast of scrambled eggs and smoked salmon with wholemeal toast instead.

POOR-QUALITY SLEEP

Sleep is essential for better exercise performance and recovery, and while drinking before bed might send you to sleep faster, it has a severe impact on sleep quality. In a study, subjects who drank alcohol just before bed did have more slow-wave sleep patterns (called delta activity), which is the period of deep sleep associated with restoration; but they also had heightened alpha-wave patterns, which your brain displays when you're awake, according to the *Alcoholism: Clinical & Experimental Research* journal. This competition between alpha and delta waves disrupts sleep, which is why you often wake up still feeling tired after drinking. And the performance impact of sleep deprivation is more pronounced in athletes, according to the journal *Sports Medicine*. The lesson? Avoid booze before bed.

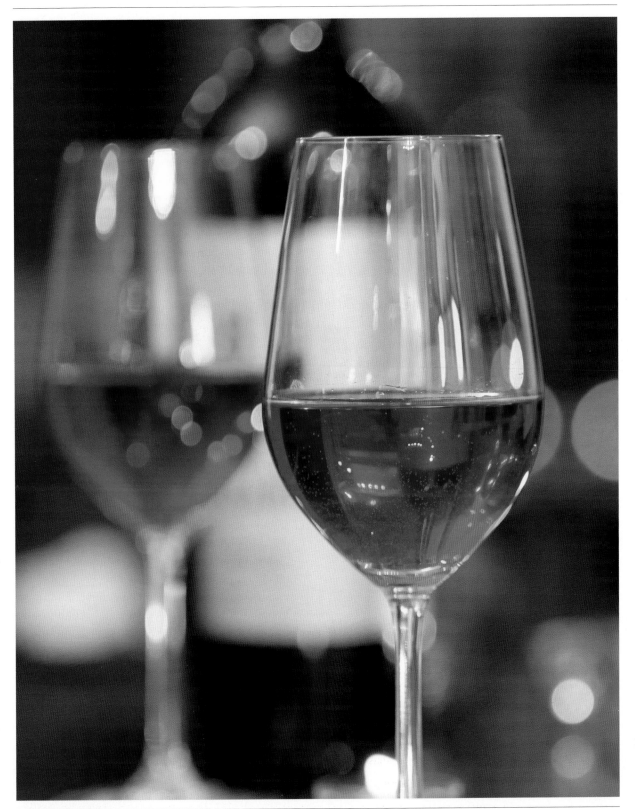

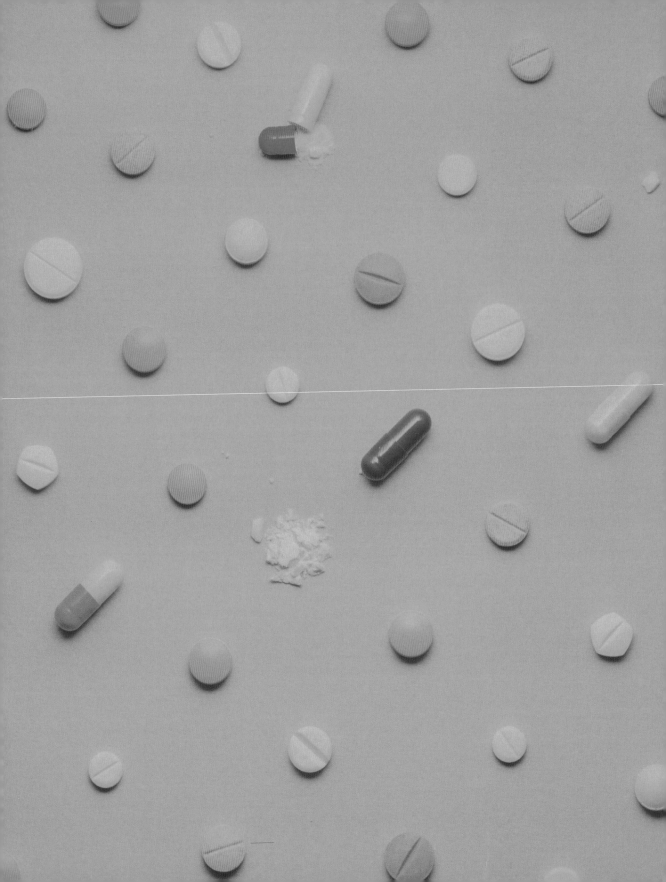

4.

Be smart with supplements

Sports supplements can be useful when you're trying to burn off body fat. They aren't magic pills – you still need to exercise and eat a healthy balanced diet – but they can make a positive difference to how you look and feel. This chapter gives you all the information you need to select the right products to support your goals.

If you've ever had an isotonic drink or popped a daily multivitamin pill, then you've taken a supplement .

While there's no single magic formula for an instant lean body – if only! – supplements can play a useful role in providing your body with all the essential vitamins, minerals and other micronutrients it needs to build muscle, burn fat and function at its best. However, they're by definition designed to *supplement* your diet, not to replace food. Eating a balanced, whole-food diet needs to be your priority, especially during the six weeks of this programme.

So think of supplements as an insurance policy to fill in any nutritional gaps that are difficult or impossible to cover with your everyday diet. Here we answer some of the most common supplement questions.

DO I REALLY NEED DIETARY SUPPLEMENTS?
Your focus should be on eating a varied and healthy diet. However, it isn't always easy to get all the essential nutrients you need every day to look, feel and perform at 100%. Intensive farming methods means produce contains less nutrients than ever before, while modern life can strip us of time and energy to prepare "proper" meals the way our parents and grandparents did, meaning we sometimes have to rely on heavily processed less healthy meal alternatives. Supplements can help fill in the gaps in your diet, but they should never be treated as the starting point for trying to improve your health and fitness. For that, training, diet and sleep should all take precedence.

ARE SUPPLEMENTS SAFE?
Most UK-based manufacturers produce only safe products, but you should always do your research into a company or a product if you have any concerns about quality or efficacy. That's because the supplement market, despite being worth more than $100 billion globally and home to almost 30,000 different products, is largely unregulated. Whereas clinical drugs must first be proven completely safe before being approved for general release, the opposite is true for dietary supplements – a product must be proved harmful before it is removed from sale.

The supplement industry is also not required to prove any of the claimed benefits associated with the product, show the safety of short- or long-term use, provide any type of quality assurance for the product, or have standardised labelling.

HOW DO I KNOW WHICH BRANDS TO TRUST?
There are now more supplement brands than ever, all trying to capitalise on the rapidly growing market. Because of the lack of industry regulation, there will be companies out there trying to make a quick buck by peddling products that, at best, have no beneficial impact and, at worst, can be detrimental to your health and fitness.

Again, your safest bet is to do your research and look into a brand or product before making a purchase. Another good rule to stick to when considering whether a product is worth buying is that if it makes a claim that sounds too good to be true, the chances are that it is. And finally, while an endorsement from a reality TV star doesn't automatically make a supplement worthless it's certainly no indication of quality.

IS IT TRUE THAT SOME BRANDS DON'T MAKE THEIR OWN PRODUCTS?
Many companies, especially new ones, don't make their own products, but simply take a white-label

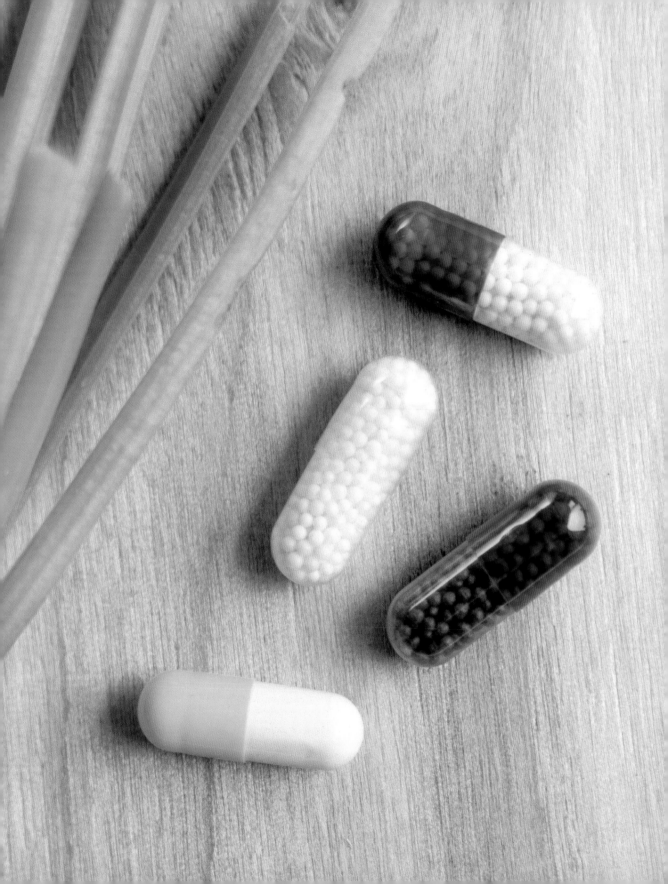

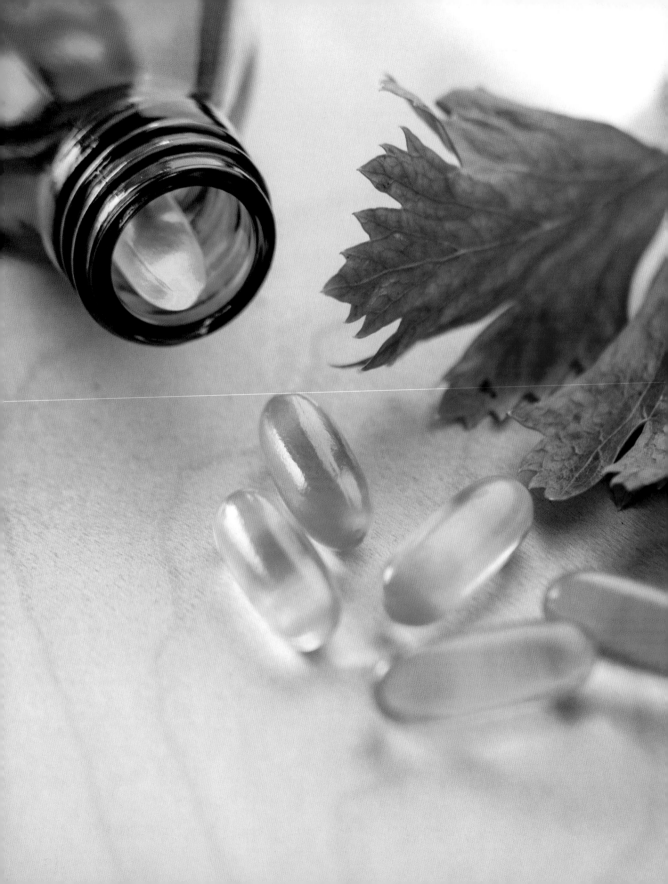

product then add their own branded packaging. This isn't necessarily a problem if the original manufacturer has high standards, as most of those based in the UK and Ireland do. However, the longer the chain from manufacturing facility to your mouth (especially if the country of origin is outside the EU) the greater the uncertainty about the quality or efficacy of the component ingredients, or what undisclosed ingredients it might contain.

ARE THERE ANY SIDE EFFECTS?
As with the consumption of any food, medicine or supplement, it is possible to experience negative side effects. Always check a product's label for substances that can cause an adverse reaction, and check the manufacturer's website for a more detailed description of potential side effects. For some supplements, such as pre-workout formulas that can contain high doses of stimulants, it's advisable to take a trial dose and monitor how you respond. Only then should you increase the dose to the manufacturer's recommendations.

CAN I USE THEM IF I FOLLOW A SPECIAL DIET?
If you are a vegetarian, vegan or follow any other restricted diet, you need to check each supplement individually to see whether it's suitable. The same goes if you have any allergies. Most reputable manufacturers detail the full ingredient breakdown of each of their products on their websites if you can't find all the information you need on a label. Failing that, you can always find their customer service helpline online and ask the company directly. If a manufacturer doesn't have enough detail displayed on it website, or is unwilling to satisfactorily answer your questions about exactly what is in one of their products, then you might want to dig a little deeper – or simply look elsewhere.

WHY ARE SOME SUPPLEMENTS SO EXPENSIVE?
Making high-quality and effective sports nutrition products isn't cheap. But, as with high-quality food, you get what you pay for. If a particular product appears to be very cheap compared with similar products from other manufacturers, it's a good idea to do a bit of online investigation into the company to find out why it's offering such cheap products before parting with your hard-earned cash.

DO I TAKE SUPPLEMENTS EVERY DAY?
It all depends on the product you're taking. Some supplements are meant to be taken daily, such as multivitamins and fish oil, because they are proven to improve general health and well-being. Others, such as whey protein powder, can also be taken as a convenient snack – even on non-training days – if you're in a hurry and don't have time to make a nutritious meal.

CAN I USE SUPPS INSTEAD OF MEALS?
Some supplements, especially in the weight loss sector, are promoted as meal-replacement products. But whether your goal is reducing body fat, building lean muscle or improving general health and fitness, fresh, whole and natural food should always be your preferred nutrition option ahead of pills, bars or shakes. These products are useful in situations where you have no alternative other than going hungry, but always remember they are called "supplements" for a good reason. Real food comes first.

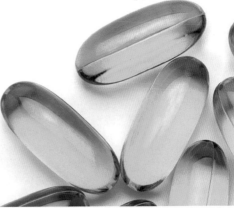

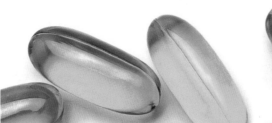

Essential supplements

If you're considering taking one, these are the first supplements you should consider

WHEY PROTEIN

WHAT IS IT? The common misconception is that whey protein powder will make you bulky but, in reality, it's just a convenient way of getting a protein hit when you can't have a proper meal. The truth is that there is nothing particularly special about whey protein. Whey is a liquid left over from milk once it has been curdled and strained to make cheese or yogurt. It isn't fundamentally different to other forms of protein, but protein powder made from whey is one of the most popular sports nutrition supplements because it is so convenient.
WHY DO I NEED IT? Anyone who is serious about getting lean fast should think about investing in a tub of high-quality whey powder. Drinking a protein shake, ideally made with whey powder and cold water or skimmed milk, within 60 minutes of the end of your training session will send amino acids straight to your muscle cells to aid your recovery.

VITAMIN D

WHAT IS IT? Vitamin D is not technically a vitamin, but a fat-soluble pre-hormone compound – one that plays an essential role in a huge number of biological functions as well as reducing the risk of certain cancers, cardiovascular disease and dementia. It is produced by your body when your skin is exposed to strong and direct sunlight, but is also found in low doses in some foods, such as fish and eggs.
WHY DO I NEED IT? If you live in the UK, or other high-latitude regions of the northern hemisphere, the chances are that you will have some level of vitamin D deficiency. One of vitamin D's main roles is to regulate the amount of calcium and phosphate in the body, which is important for your bones and many other cells. Supplementation can keep your levels in the ideal range to help prevent these problems, but be aware that taking high doses can deplete levels of other essential nutrients, including vitamin K.

MAGNESIUM

WHAT IS IT? The chemical element magnesium is an essential trace element. This means every single cell in your body needs magnesium ions to function, because they're involved in the production of energy, while hundreds of enzymes require its presence to work optimally. Nuts, green leafy vegetables and wholegrains are the best dietary sources.
WHY DO I NEED IT? The UK recommended daily intake for magnesium is 270mg for women. But 68% of Americans not hitting their daily target, according to the US Department of Agriculture, and it's likely that this is replicated in the UK given our similar diets and lifestyles. Magnesium is needed for central nervous system function and muscle contractions, both of which are a big part of training, and exercise can deplete your levels. Supplementation is wise if you work out intensively and often.

MULTIVITAMIN

WHAT IS IT? Exactly what is sounds like: a tablet or capsule that contains a high percentage of the recommended daily intake of the vitamins and minerals your body needs to function at its best.
WHY DO I NEED IT? If you are eating a natural and varied whole-food diet, you should be getting all the vitamins and minerals you need. However, with the best will in the world, it's not always convenient or even possible to eat a diet consisting exclusively of natural unprocessed foods, and sometimes we all resort to the mass-produced factory foods that dominate our supermarket aisles. Besides, soil and air pollution and increasing pesticide use mean that even many natural foods now have lower levels of nutrients than ever before. A daily multivitamin can act as a good insurance policy to ensure you hit your daily target of essential nutrients.

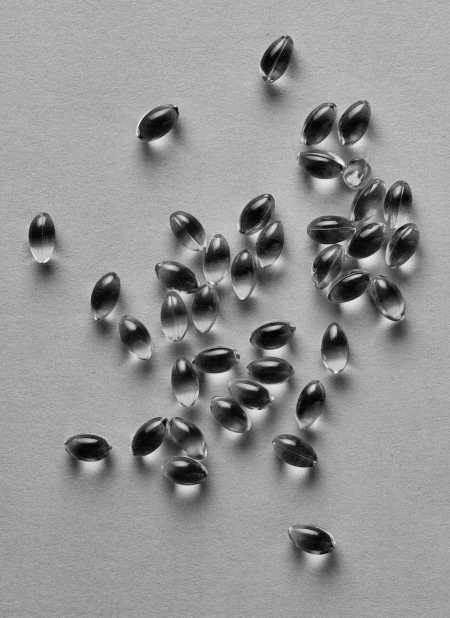

OMEGA 3

WHAT IS IT? Omega 3 is an essential fatty acid, which means that our bodies can't manufacture it so we need to consume it directly in our diet. It is found in high concentrations in oily fish, especially those from cold-water climates.
WHY DO I NEED IT? Omega 3 is crucial for healthy metabolic function, and adequate intake provides a whole host of other immediate and long-term health benefits, including aiding fat loss, better mental function and performance, and reduced inflammation, as well as reducing the risk of cardiovascular disease, certain cancers and mental health disorders. The consumption of fish is an important component of a healthy and balanced diet. If you're not getting the recommended two weekly portions of fish (one oily and one non-oily) – and the chances are you're not because the UK average is only one-third of a portion a week – then you should consider supplementation.

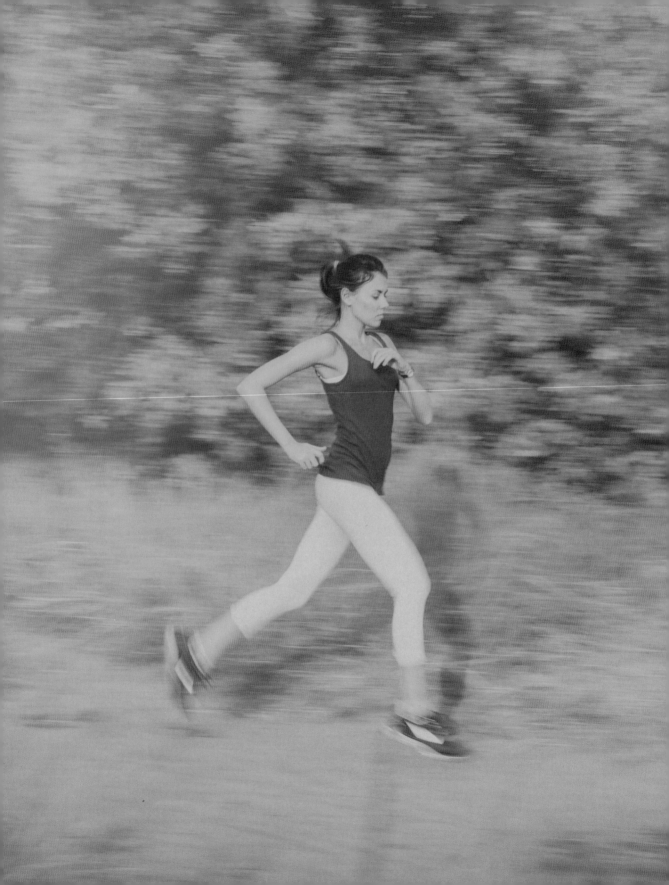

5.

Become a cardio queen

Cardio exercise is in many ways the easiest form of training there is – just jump on a bike, lace up your shoes or dive in and away you go! But if you're going to use cardio as an effective fat loss tool, there's a little more to know. This chapter shows you how to make the most of your sessions to maximise the fat burn.

Cardio training can be great for your physical and mental health and well-being – that's not in doubt. But to make running, cycling and swimming sessions into legitimate fat loss workouts, you need to take a smarter approach to training. And that means you need to make your cardio sessions, whether in the gym or outside, short and intense to elevate your heart rate, as well as pushing yourself hard enough to ensure you leave your comfort zone well behind you. The best way to do this is though high-intensity interval training (HIIT), which we'll explain in more detail in the next chapter, but first here's why longer forms of cardio training aren't great for fat loss.

If you've tried and failed to lose weight before, the chances are you started doing more running or cycling, especially longer-distance jogs or rides. But while steady-state cardio – which is when you run, cycle or swim at a consistent and comfortable intensity for a significant amount of time – has many health benefits, maximising fat loss isn't one of them. That's because this type of endurance-based exercise doesn't push your heart, lungs and muscles hard enough to significantly initiate the process by which your body is forced to start tapping into fat cells to release fuel for energy.

Many people often eat loads of pasta and other carbohydrates after a session to replenish their energy, which –as we explained in our fat loss myths on p8 – can mean you're consuming more calories than you just burned. And that's not an effective way to lose fat because you need to burn more calories than you consume every day to force your body to give up its fat stores.

So if you love nothing better than to head out for a good old cardio session but want to turn those sessions into fat-blasting workouts, you need to follow the advice in this chapter.

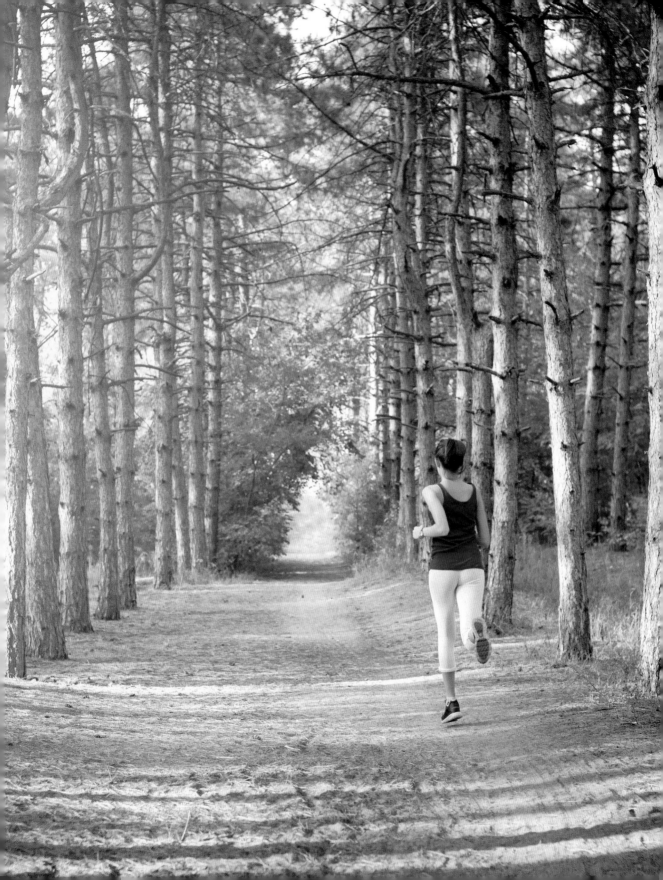

Crush your cardio

Follow these strategies for every cardio training session if you want to burn maximum fat

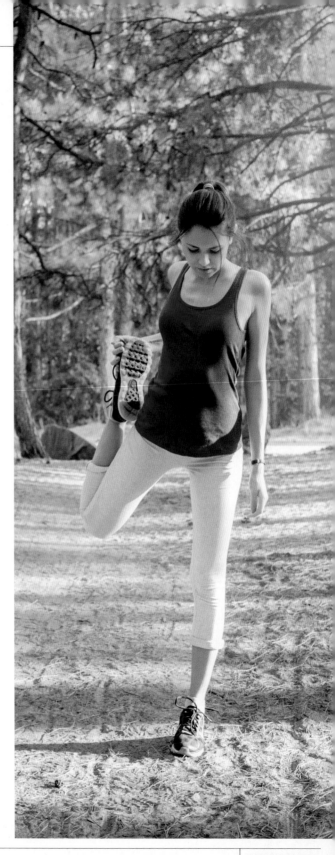

WARM UP WELL

Before you begin any session, you need to thoroughly warm up your cardiovascular system and your major muscles to prepare for the intense work ahead to reduce your risk of injury. Do 10 minutes of gentle activity, gradually increasing the intensity, until you feel warmer and a little out of breath.

STRETCH DYNAMICALLY

For decades we were told that static holds and stretches were the best way to prepare the muscles for exercise. In fact, more recent and thorough research has established that forcing them into held stretches when they are cold and tight makes them weaker and primes them for injury. Instead do some dynamic stretching – think high knee raises and similar moves – as part of your warm-up.

UP THE INTENSITY

Once you're warmed up you can start the session. Remember the key is to exercise in short, intense bursts of effort to raise your heart rate and fire up your muscles for a double fat-burning effect. Studies have proven that well-executed interval sessions will both decrease body-fat levels and increase lean muscle mass. Whatever activity you are doing, work up to doing all-out effort sets of lasting 10 to 30 seconds any longer than that and you won't be training at your maximum intensity.

KEEP RESTS BRIEF
To keep your heart rate elevated for as much of the session as possible, keep rest periods between your exertions short. For instance, if you are doing 20-second all-out sprints, you can go at a gentler recovery pace for 40 seconds between them, keeping each set to a round minute and making it easier to be consistent with your effort levels throughout the session. If you're doing sprints in a park, then you could sprint for 60-80m, then walk back slowly to the start as a recovery before repeating.

DON'T OVERDO IT
A cardio interval session can be very taxing on your heart, lungs, central nervous system and muscles, so it's important that you don't overdo it, especially if you are new to this training approach. If so, keep sessions short – 20-25 minutes including your warm-up is fine – to gradually get your body used to the demands of these workouts. There's no need to do a long interval session, because you should do each work set with all-out effort so you will become fatigued quickly. Keeping these sessions short and intense is the key to making them successful.

DO A WARM-DOWN
As well as warming up beforehand you need to warm down afterwards so that your body can gradually move back to rest mode from activity mode. Around five to 10 minutes of exercise – jogging if you've been sprinting, or easier laps if you've been swimming – is enough to bring your heart rate back down and flush waste products from your muscles. Gradually reduce the intensity until your heart rate is back to its normal resting level.

Intense inspiration
Three interval session ideas to get you started

Bike sprints
Walk into any gym and you're likely to see someone on a stationary bike, flicking through a magazine or scrolling down their phone while pedalling. This workout (and the other two cardio sessions here) is basically the opposite of that approach. Sit on the bike at the correct height – with a slight bend in your knee when the pedal is at the bottom – and warm up for five minutes at a comfortable pace. Then, every minute on the minute, do 20 seconds of sprinting followed by 40 seconds at recovery pace. Repeat for a total of 10 minutes. Then try not to fall off the bike.

Deadmills
Get on the treadmill and warm up for five minutes. Then turn the machine off. That's right, the treadmill becomes the deadmill. Stand on the stationary belt, holding on to the support bars by the machine's screen or panel, and lean slightly forward from the hips. Then take big powerful strides forward to get the belt moving until you have built up enough speed to start sprinting. Go all-out for 15 to 20 seconds, then slow down until the belt is stationary again. Rest for 45-60 seconds and repeat. Aim to do eight to 10 rounds.

Row repeats
Put the damper setting at 6-8 to make sure each stroke is sufficiently difficult, then position yourself correctly and safely on the rower with feet securely fastened and an overhand grip on the bar. Make sure the screen is on and that the time and distance data are clearly visible. Row for five minutes at a comfortable pace, then row for 250m as fast as possible while maintaining proper rowing form. Recover at your comfortable pace for 60 seconds, then row another 250m at maximum effort. Repeat this pattern for a total of five all-out 250m rows.

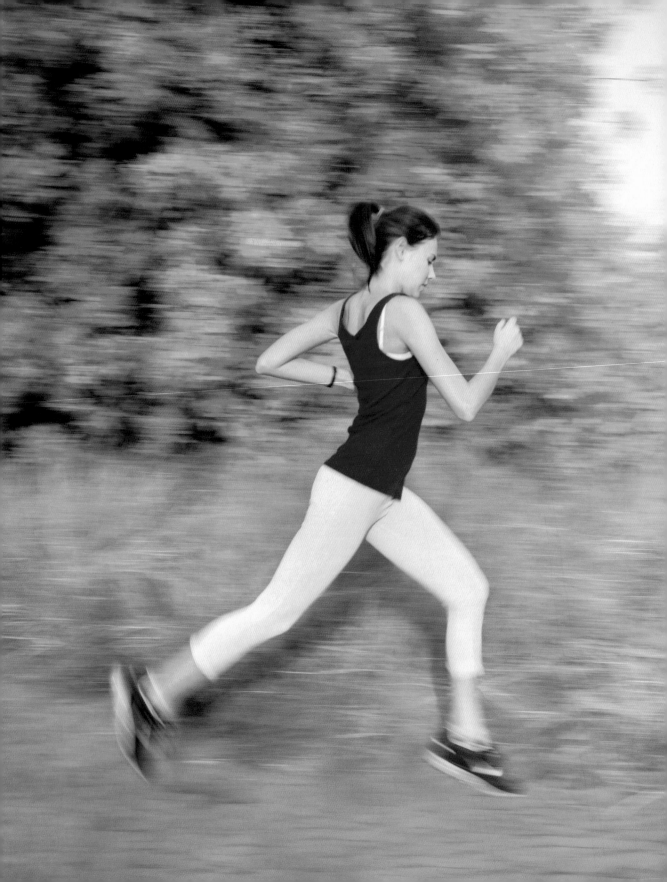

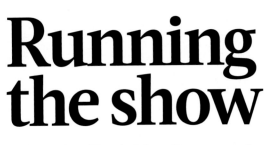

Running the show

Regular running will burn body fat and improve general feelings of physical and mental health and well-being. Here's all you need to know about becoming a better runner

Look at any professional runner, whether that's a sprinter or marathon runner, and you'll see that – despite their different disciplines and body shapes – the one thing they all have in common is that they don't carry much body fat. And if you want to build a leaner and more athletic physique, you need to think and train more like the pros. Over the following pages we explain the key areas in which you need to improve to strip away body fat while becoming a stronger and better runner. First up are some pro performance tips, followed by advice on nutrition, recovery and injury prevention, as well as tips on how to buy the right running shoes for your goal.

Performance tips

Make your runs more effective with these tips from elite runner and coach Shaun Dixon

TRAIN FASTER

Dedicated speed sessions burn body fat efficiently and make you a faster runner. They do so by improving your neural pathways (the way your brain communicates with your muscles) so that your muscles contract quicker and harder for more power output per stride and greater running economy. What's more, they'll also get you used to dealing with lactic acid so you can run faster for longer.

Intervals should last no longer than 90 seconds so you can maintain an intensity of around 85% of your maximum effort throughout. Rest between each interval should be three to four times the length of the drill, to allow you to maintain sprint quality. Start with 10 reps of around 40 seconds. If you find you're slowing during a sprint, end the session because only quality reps count when you want to get leaner and faster. Another benefit, although it won't feel good at the time, is that you will experience a significant lactic acid build-up through these drills, and the better you are at tolerating lactic acid the quicker you'll run. Make sure you warm up thoroughly first.

WORK ON TECHNIQUE

Without good technique you'll never run the most efficient session possible, and you'll also increase your risk of injury. For the correct posture, stand tall by holding your hips high and lean forwards slightly, putting your weight on your toes. You should be able to draw a straight line through your ears, shoulders and hips. You want to minimise lateral movement at your shoulders and hips, and minimise torso movement by lowering your shoulders and driving your arms backwards from the shoulder joint.

You also want to keep a high turnover of steps – your goal is to spend less time in contact with the ground. That's because long, heavy strides are much less efficient than shorter and faster strides that include only a brief contact with the ground.

DO A STRIDES SESSION

This is a staple session elite runners use to improve neuromuscular pathways and get the muscles firing faster. After a short easy-pace run, find a flat uninterrupted path or pavement between 80 and 100m in length and run fast and smoothly for the entire length. You don't need to go "eyeballs out" as you would for a HIIT session but aim for between 85% and 90% of your maximum effort while staying as focused and relaxed as possible. Run six to eight reps, with a slow jog or walk back to your starting position after each one. Do a strides session once or twice a fortnight.

RUN FOR THE HILLS

Hill runs are the simplest form of speed session because they're easy to plan, they don't require much thinking and – while they tend to be tough – they're over quickly. Uphill sessions are great for the glutes, get your heart rate high for fat loss benefits and challenge your body's ability to process lactic acid, a key factor in improving speed. Find a steep hill, run up it for 30 to 45 seconds fast, then walk back down and repeat for six to eight reps.

GO DOWNHILL FAST

Alternatively you could run down the hill, a strategy used by Kenyan runners to improve foot turnover because you have to keep your feet moving fast to prevent the heavy jarring of your joints. Find a hill with a slight incline. At the top stand tall, then lean forwards as you start to run. Pick up your heels quickly and employ short, fast steps, making your contact with the ground quick and light. Try six to eight downhill reps of 30 seconds, jogging back up to the top after each one.

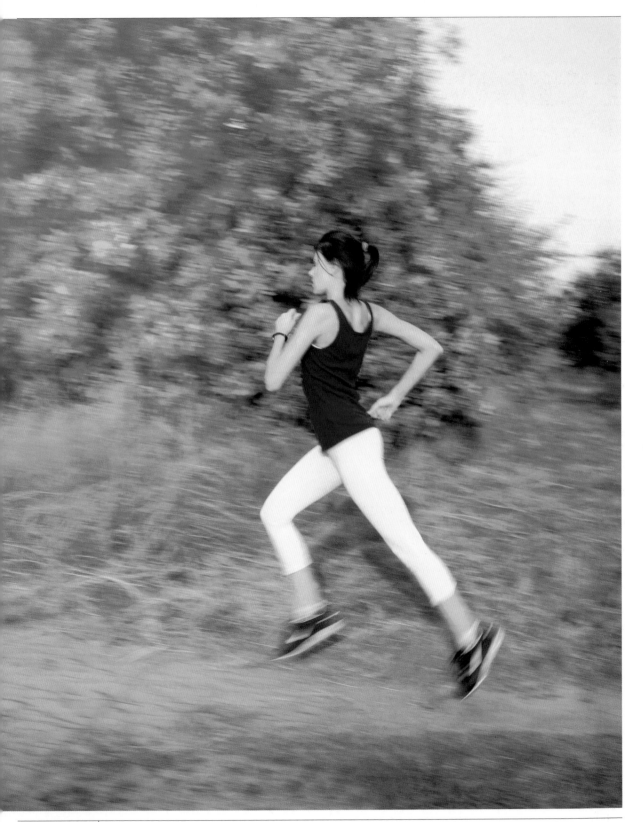

Beat injury

Build an injury-proof body with advice from biomechanics consultant Travis Allan, who has worked with Olympic triathletes and elite athletes

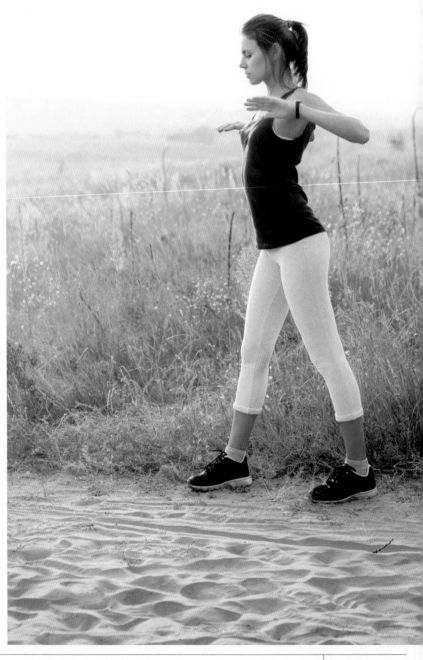

If you're following a training plan like the one in this book injury is a sure way to mess it up. So it's advisable to take preventative action by doing some injury-proofing exercises, focusing on your feet. Runners often don't think about foot exercises, but they're important because if your foot isn't hitting the ground properly you can develop common problems like runner's knee or connective tissue pain.

The drills here are "prehab" exercises that will improve your capacity to absorb the shock of each stride and prevent joint stress and strain. Perform them in order, either before a run or on non-running days. Some of the movements are subtle so to get the full benefit, follow the form guides and concentrate on the precise movements.

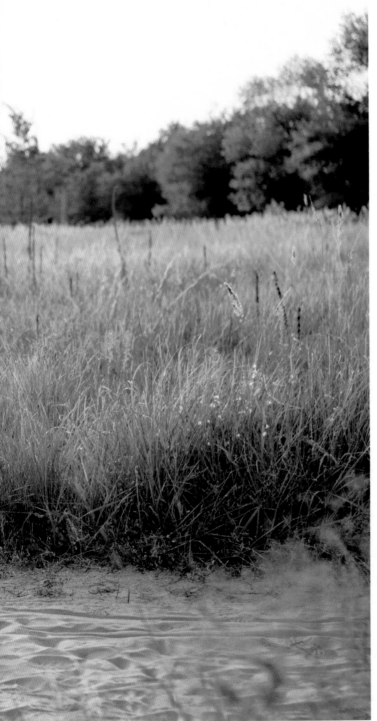

FOOT EVERSION

Lie on your back with your knees bent and both feet flat on the floor. Secure an exercise band around your mid-foot (not your toes) on both feet so that there is a small amount of tension in the band when your feet are roughly shoulder-width apart. On one foot, tilt the heel and big toe inwards slightly, then sweep your foot outwards across the floor to create a stretch in the band. You'll know you're doing it correctly if you feel a muscle contraction in the outside of your lower leg. Hold that position for a count of 6sec. Come back to the start position for 6-10sec and repeat that six times. Then do the same on the other foot.

FOOT INVERSION

Lie on your back with your knees bent and both feet flat on the floor. Secure an exercise band around your mid-foot on both feet and cross one foot over the other. Let your heel roll outwards, but don't tilt it so far that you're on the side of your foot. Then sweep your foot inwards until you feel a muscle contraction on the inside of your lower leg. Hold that position for a count of 6sec. Come back to the start position for 6-10sec and repeat that six times. Then do the same on the other foot.

PLANTAR FLEXION

Lie on your back with your knees bent and both feet flat on the floor. Take one foot back and place the top of that foot behind your other heel. Gently push the forefoot of your front foot into the ground, rotate your foot inwards slightly and pull it back in towards your other foot so you feel your calf muscle engage. Hold that position for a count of 6sec, rest for 6-10sec and repeat that six times. Then do the same on the other foot.

DORSIFLEXION

Lie on your back with your knees bent and both feet flat on the floor. Flex the toes on both feet to raise them off the floor but try to avoid pulling your whole foot off the floor. Hold that position for a count of 6sec. Come back to the start position for 6-10sec and repeat that six times.

Sample sessions

Burn more body fat faster by finding the right running session for you

INTERVAL SESSION

An interval session is a structured run during which you alternate between different training intensities, typically exercising at a set pace for a certain amount of time. So a session might switch between running at low intensity for a minute, medium intensity for a minute, then high intensity for 30 seconds, then move back down through the gears and then go up them again. This type of session is very effective at getting your heart and lungs working hard to increase the amount of oxygen going to your muscles, increasing the rate at which you burn calories both during your run and in the hours afterwards as your body recovers.

FARTLEK SESSION

Fartlek, which is Swedish for "speed play", is a training approach where you alternate between periods of intense effort and speed and slower periods of recovery. Unlike an interval session, though, it is not structured so you switch between training intensities as and when you feel like it. A good example would be a road running session where every time you pass a lamppost you increase or decrease your effort level, alternating between high and low as you run. The switching of effort levels places demands on both your aerobic (with oxygen) and anaerobic (without oxygen) energy systems, which is an effective way to burn body fat faster.

HILL SESSION

Hill running is a highly effective way to torch fat, improve leg strength and test your cardiovascular system. But be warned: these are extremely hard sessions and you need to follow a few simple rules to make them as effective as possible and protect yourself against injury. First you need to find a hill. It doesn't matter how steep it is because you simply reduce the distance you run up it the steeper it is. After a thorough warm-up, run your predetermined uphill distance as quickly as possible, then walk back down and repeat. You can do this session for time, or for a set number of sprints.

SPEED SESSION

A speed session is designed to improve the top speed at which you can run. In many respects they are a bit like hill sessions except you do them on a flat surface – the pavement, the track or even a treadmill. Warming up thoroughly first is essential to prepare your body for such a highly intense session. You then sprint for a set distance – 60m to 100m is recommended – as fast as you can, maintaining good posture and form. You then rest for up to two minutes and repeat for a set number of sprints (up to about eight is ideal). However, if your top speed suddenly declines, end the session – only quality sprints count.

STEADY-STATE SESSION

This type of session is exactly what it sounds like – a longer run in which your speed is consistent throughout. Training like this forms a key part of any marathon or long-distance challenge because it is one of best strategies to improve endurance. As mentioned previously, while long steady-state sessions do burn calories, there are better and more effective ways to tap into body fat stores when running, including all four of the other sessions described here. However, long cardio sessions do have other positive health outcomes, including better muscular endurance, better cardiovascular function, and improved mood and other mental health benefits.

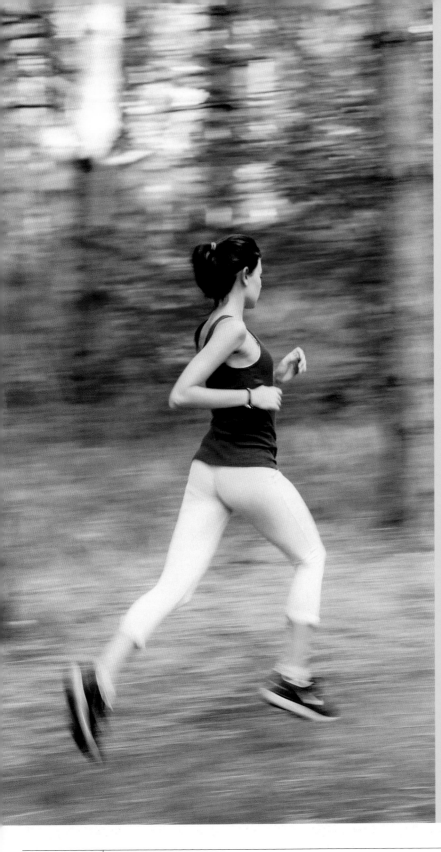

Hit the road

Try these three cardio sessions

INTERVAL SESSION

Do this session on the road, in the park or on a treadmill.
Warm-up 5min
Low-intensity effort 2min
Medium-intensity effort 2min
High-intensity effort 30sec
Medium-intensity effort 2min
Low-intensity effort 1min
Medium-intensity effort 1min
High-intensity effort 30sec
Medium-intensity effort 1min
High-intensity effort 30sec
Medium-intensity effort 1min
High-intensity effort 30sec
Medium-intensity effort 1min
High-intensity effort 30sec
Medium-intensity effort 2min
Low-intensity effort 2min
Warm-down 5min

HILL SESSION

Do this session on a hill that has
an incline of at least 40m or on a
treadmill with an adjustable incline.
Warm-up 5min
Hill sprint 60m (or 10sec)
Recover 2min
Repeat for a total of 8 reps, then
do a 5min warm-down.

SPEED SESSION

Do this session on the road, in
the park or on a treadmill.
Warm-up 5min
Sprint 50-100m
Recovery 2-3min
Repeat for a total of 8 reps, then
do a 5min warm-down.

Nutrition

Help your body burn fat faster with these nutrition rules for running from Renee McGregor, a performance and clinical dietitian and the author of *Training Food*

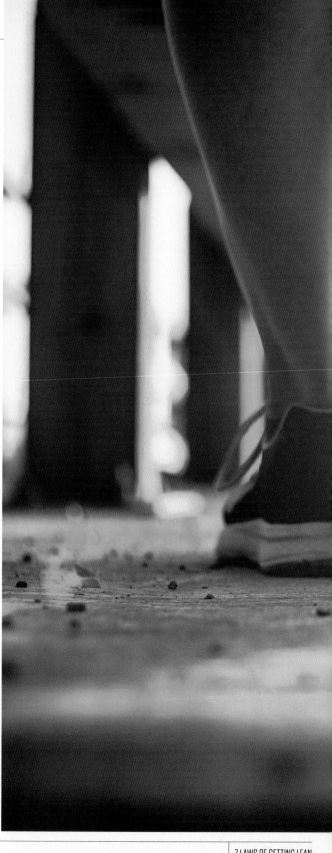

RUN HUNGRY

Try running in a fasted state for slow to moderate runs lasting up to 45 minutes, which means not eating in the two hours before setting out, or running first thing before breakfast. This improves your body's ability to tap into fat stores for fuel, which makes you a more efficient runner, as well as helping you lose weight. If you're new to running you need to work up gradually to training in a fully fasted state, because it can suppress your immune system if you don't give your body time to adjust.

REFUEL AFTER RUNNING

While running in a fasted state can offer many performance benefits, it means refuelling correctly immediately after your run is even more important. Your post-run meal will aid recovery so if you do run fasted, it's vital to eat a proper meal – containing carbs for energy replacement and a good source of protein for muscle repair – as soon as possible.

EAT THE RIGHT CARBS

For any run lasting more than 60 minutes some easily digestible carbs – a smoothie, banana on toast or porridge with honey – in the hour or two before you start will improve performance. You should also ensure you eat enough carbs over the 24 hours before the run so your muscles' glycogen stores are filled. This is essential for longer, more intense runs so that your body has all the easy-to-use fuel it needs to perform consistently well for the whole session.

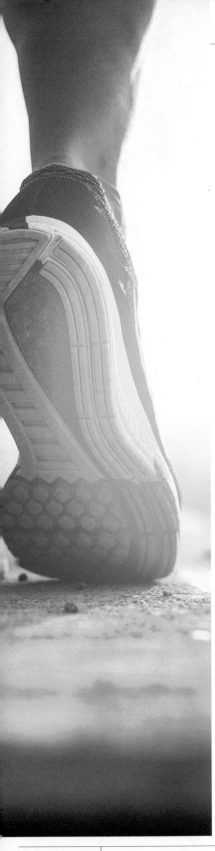

Footwear

Run in the right trainers to get more out of every single session

Specialist running trainers fall into one of five groups: motion control, cushioned, stability, lightweight and trail. Pick the right pair for your feet and training needs with this guide from the experts at specialist running shop Runners Need (runnersneed.com).

CHOOSE THE RIGHT TYPE

Consider where you're going to be running and buy shoes that will be suitable for the terrain. If most of your training is off-road, then road shoes with built-up heels are unsuitable because you will be less stable and could turn an ankle. Similarly, a pair of trail running shoes with deeply studded outsoles will be very uncomfortable on paved roads, because the studs will press into the soles of your feet.

SELECT SMARTER SOCKS

You should always wear the socks that you intend to run in when you go for a shoe fitting. The thickness of your sock can make a big difference to the fit and feel of your shoe, particularly as your feet expand in the heat. Runners should wear running-specific socks because these have extra padding across the ball of the foot, the toe and the heel area. This extra padding reduces impact and protects important areas that can blister. There's also usually padding or a tighter area through the arch to allow the shoe to fit more closely and add better arch support.

GET GAIT ANALYSIS

A free gait analysis service is offered at many specialist running stores. You'll be videoed or observed by an in-store expert while running on a treadmill for a couple of minutes, and then the expert will use the video and/or their experience to assess your foot plant, stride and running pattern. This information can then be used to find the best shoe for you.

GO FOR A TRIAL RUN

Buying your running shoes is a big investment, so you should always test any shoes properly before buying them. Padding around on a carpet in the shop certainly won't replicate how the shoes will feel when you're running in them. Instead, you should "road test" them on an in-store treadmill.

DON'T WEAR THEM OUT

Your running shoes will take a great deal of pounding across a wide range of surfaces and in all weathers, so they will need to be replaced fairly frequently. Generally you should replace a pair after 500-600 miles (800-960km). Exactly how often you need to buy new shoes will depend on your weight, running style and choice of terrain, but avoid trying to squeeze a few extra weeks out of shoes that are evidently worn out, because the shoes won't give you the protection you need and that will increase the chances of injury.

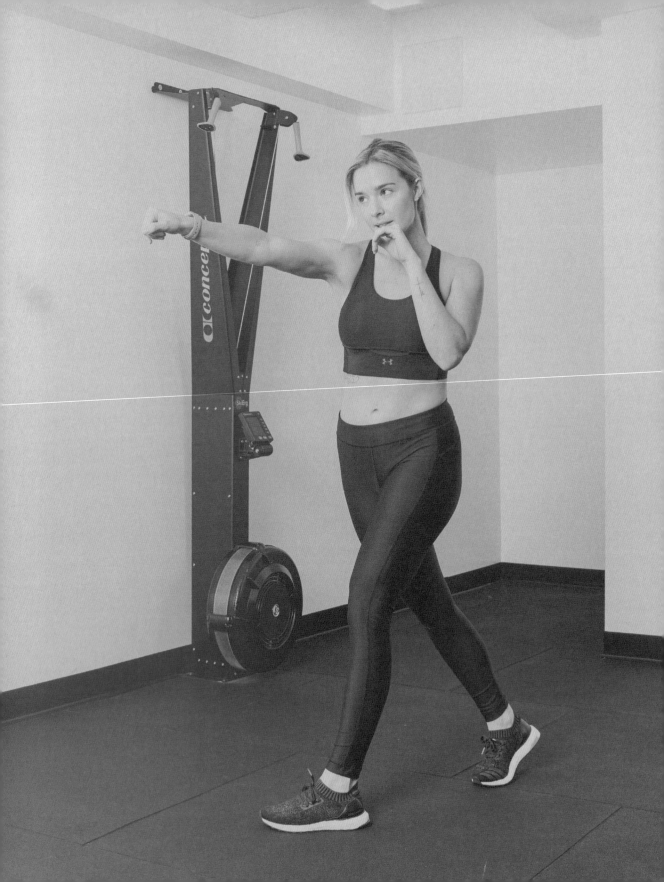

6.
Harness HIIT power

High-intensity interval training offers a highly effective (and highly sweaty!) fast track to fat loss. This chapter tells you everything you need to know about building fat loss workouts, as well as detailing a step-by-step plan that will transform your body in six weeks. Just remember to use it in conjunction with our nutrition tips.

High-intensity interval training, or HIIT, has become popular in recent years and – unlike some fitness fads – there's a lot of evidence to support its effectiveness as a training system. One benefit that you don't need a degree in exercise science to understand is that HIIT workouts tend to be short. Most of the sessions in this chapter come in at around 20 minutes.

For most people, a short HIIT workout is a far more attractive option than spending an hour in the gym or pounding the pavements endlessly. In fact, in a recent study published in the journal *Topics In Spinal Cord Injury Rehabilitation*, researchers found that when they asked subjects to list their barriers to exercise, "lack of time" was the most common response. Similarly, if motivation is a problem, HIIT could be the answer because the intense, dynamic and challenging nature of the workouts mean that they are always engaging – you'll get tired, sure, but you won't be bored.

Some solid scientific data backs up the idea of using HIIT for fat loss. One study, published in the *Journal Of Sports Medicine And Physical Fitness*, compared conventional gym training with HIIT training and found that "HIIT resulted in significantly greater reduction in both abdominal girth and visceral adiposity compared with conventional training". Visceral adiposity means fat stored around the organs, too much of which can bring serious health problems. The same study also found that HIIT had a positive impact on total body fat, hand grip strength, sprint endurance, jumping ability and flexibility.

There are other benefits you get from doing a HIIT workout that involves resistance training (ie shifting weight, including bodyweight moves), as opposed to just cardiovascular activity such as running. Pure cardio is useful, but it shouldn't be the only kind of training you do because resistance training will improve your strength and also your body composition (improving your ratio of muscle to body fat). Do that and you'll usher in a host of other health benefits such as increased life expectancy and reduced risk of heart disease.

Of course, just as one type of training won't give you everything you're looking for, this chapter shouldn't be used in isolation. Combine it with the previous five chapters and you'll make significant changes to your body in a short space of time – and when you're finished with this chapter, you can add the final piece to your fat loss puzzle with the advice in our final muscle-toning chapter.

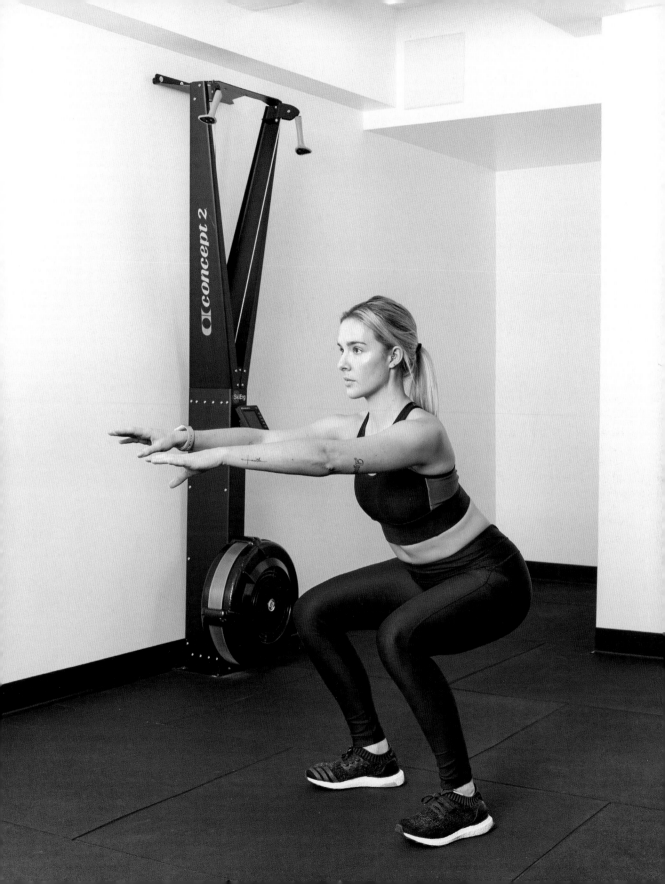

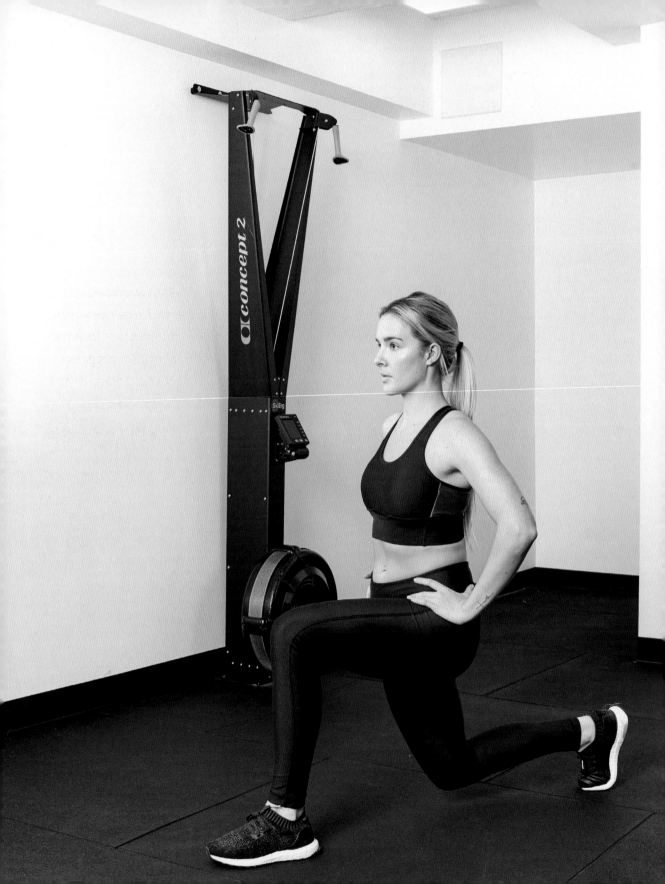

Fat loss training FAQ

Fat loss might start in the kitchen, but it accelerates in the gym. By working at a high intensity and building some muscle, you'll torch fat as well as ramping up your metabolism, making burning fat faster and easier. The plan in this chapter gives you workouts to follow but with the advice below, you'll be able to create your own sessions too so you can continue to make progress after you finish the plan or adjust your training according to your needs.

What's best for fat loss – weights or cardio?
Both work – if you do them properly. Traditional jogging-style cardio isn't ideal for fat loss, because it can elevate your stress hormones and make you hungry, so short, intense efforts are better. Whatever tool you're using for fat loss, the principles are the same: keep your heart rate high and the rests short.

If I do fat loss workouts, can I eat what I want?
No. Sorry! Training might give you a bit of leeway with an otherwise-strict diet, but even an hour in the gym's easily undone with a whipped-cream mochaccino. Stay on top of what you eat, although you shouldn't beat yourself up over the occasional slip-up.

How often can I do a fat loss workout?
If you're going to do high-intensity sessions, three or four times a week is a sensible upper limit - you'd be better off spending any extra time on restorative sessions such a yoga, or even just shopping for food and cooking. Want more work? Go for a nice long walk: it'll burn calories without over-stressing your system.

Do I need to do any other type of training?
If you're doing mobility movements like yoga as part of your fat loss, you're probably fine. Mobility and toning work will alleviate your risk of age-related disease, and if you focus on muscle tone then you'll look better once you've stripped away the fat.

How long do my fat loss workouts need to be?
Good news: fat loss workouts are some of the shortest you can do while still making great progress. Even 15 minutes is enough – do a quick warm-up, then hit a training interval (eg 30 seconds of work and 30 seconds of rest) for ten minutes, and you're done.

6-week belly blast

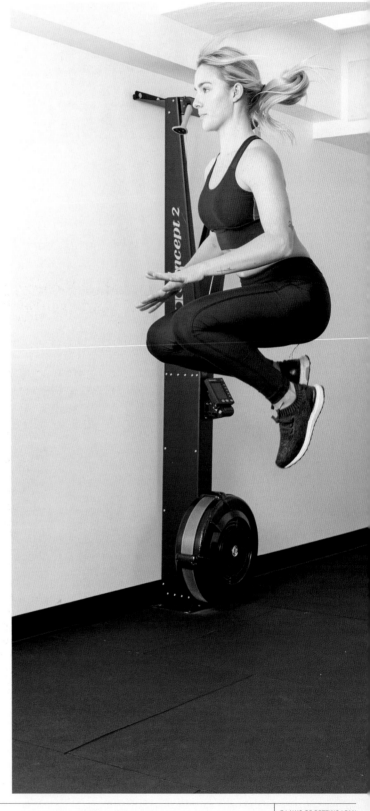

How much of a difference do you think you can really make to how you look and feel in six weeks? The good news: a lot. The less good, more realistic news is that you can only make that change if you follow an effective plan and work hard. We've done the first bit for you but the second element is entirely dependent on your commitment. So before you start your six-week fat loss transformation, you may want to go back to p10 and re-read the chapter on improving your mindset to make sure you know both how to start this particular fitness journey and how to stick with it. You also need to make sure you follow our nutrition advice alongside the workout plan if you want to get the most impressive result possible.

HOW DOES THE PLAN WORK?

It's simple: you complete four circuit workouts a week for six weeks. Each circuit is a whole-body workout and you do the same circuits each week but change the work and rest variables to make them progressively harder. You don't need any kit so you can do it either in the gym or at home. It's advisable to take rest days between workout days – but they're not so taxing that it's essential to do so.

WHY DOES THE PLAN WORK?

There are several key reasons why the plan works. Each circuit is a whole-body workout, so they challenge every major muscle group in your body. The workouts also get your heart rate high, so you'll burn a lot of calories both during and after your sessions. And the plan gets harder each week, so you'll keep progressing throughout the plan.

WHAT IF I'M A BEGINNER?

The plan is beginner-friendly because it doesn't require lots of fancy kit and all the exercises are achievable if you're in good health. If you're a beginner, start steadily and gradually increase the intensity. You should aim to complete as many reps as you can in each work period so you'll need to pick a tempo that's appropriate for your fitness levels. This might take a session or two to work out, so allow yourself a bit of time to get to grips with the physical demands.

WHAT DO I DO AFTER SIX WEEKS?

The first thing you should do is give yourself a big pat on your, by now, lean and toned back. Completing any training plan takes a lot of work and dedication, so focus first on getting to the end of the programme. Once you've done that, you can use the information at the end of this section to decide on what would be the best next move. Your main options: doing it again but with longer work periods; doing the muscle-toning plan in the next chapter; or taking on an entirely new fitness challenge.

Week 1
Circuit 1

The circuits in this routine target different body parts with each exercise. This means that you work hard during the allotted time for each exercise but you are also able to recover sufficiently to make it all the way through the session. This makes your cardiovascular system work harder because your work rate can remain high, and your heart also has to pump blood to the part of the body targeted by the exercise. There's a bias towards lower-body exercises because they tend to give you more bang for your fat-burning buck. The session finishes with a dynamic abs move and a static one so you target your abs – helping you add definition to your tummy muscles – as well as losing fat.

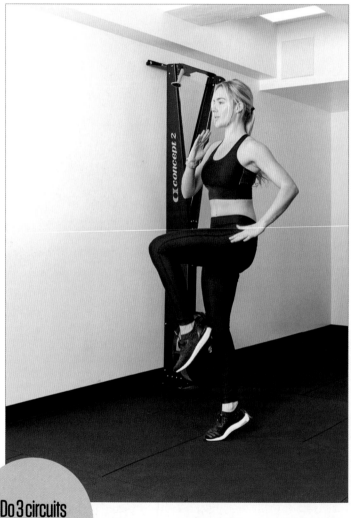

Do 3 circuits in total

EXERCISE	TIME	REST
1 Split squat	30sec	30sec
2 Punches	30sec	30sec
3 Lunge	30sec	30sec
4 Run on the spot	30sec	30sec
5 Mountain climber	30sec	30sec
6 Straight-arm plank	30sec	2min

1 Split squat

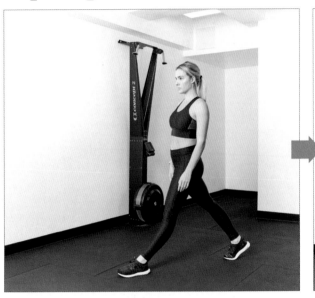

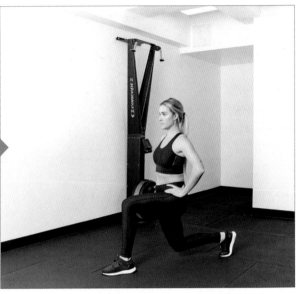

HOW Take a step forwards into a staggered stance, then simultaneously bend both knees to lower towards the floor. Press back up to the start to complete the rep.

WHY This is the most accessible way of starting a squat or lunge movement but it is also physically demanding enough to give you a fat loss benefit.

2 Punches

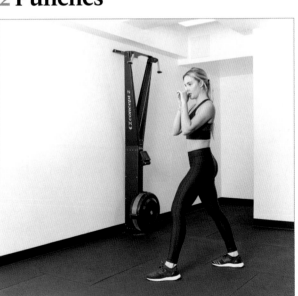

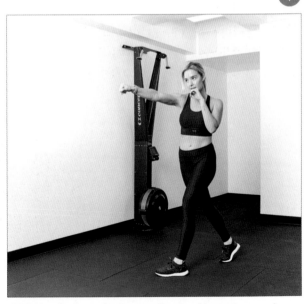

HOW Stand with your fists at your shoulders, then throw alternate punches, rotating your wrists as you throw the punch so that your palms face down when your arm is straight.

WHY You don't need to be a professional boxer to get the benefits of boxing training. This fun move will tone your arms and get your heart rate high.

3 Lunge

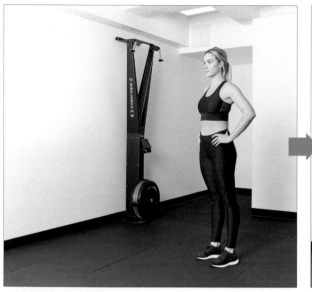

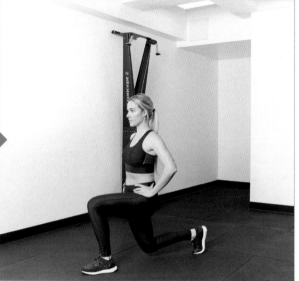

HOW Stand tall, then take a big stride forwards and bend both knees simultaneously. Press through your front heel to return to the start. Swap sides with each rep.

WHY The lunge is a one-sided move so it will help you to build a balanced body. It's also an excellent move for toning your glutes.

4 Run on the spot

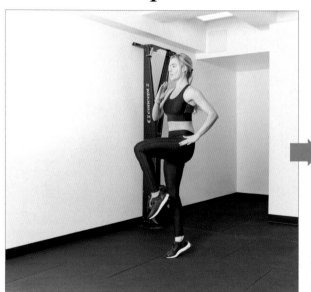

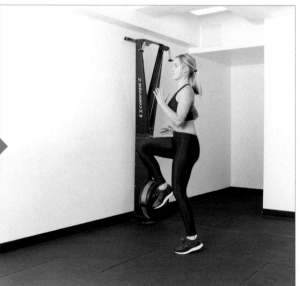

HOW Run on the spot, aiming to raise your knees high, swinging your arms with your elbows bent at approximately 90 degrees.

WHY This is a safe and simple way of getting your heart rate up, which will maximise calorie burn, and it will also improve your balance and coordination.

5 Mountain climber

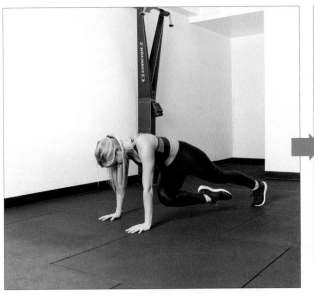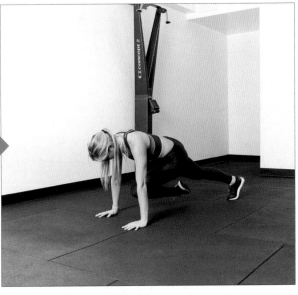

HOW Get into the top of a press-up position, then jump one foot forwards so it is under your chest. Simultaneously jump that foot back to the start and the other forwards.

WHY This is a deceptively tough exercise that will test your upper-body strength and your cardio fitness, while also toning your side abs.

6 Straight-arm plank

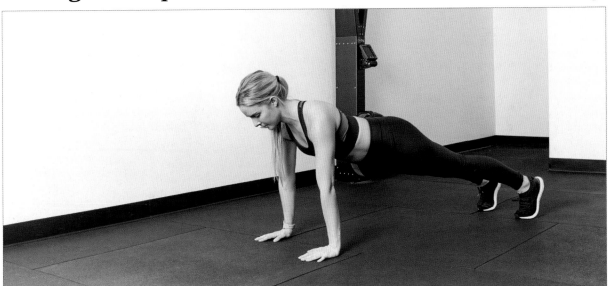

HOW Make sure your body is in a straight line from head to heels. Your hands should be directly below your shoulders. Hold the position and don't let your hips sag.

WHY The straight-arm version of the plank is more accessible than the standard version (see p79), which will allow you to get familiar with controlling your core muscles.

Circuit 2

The circuits in your second routine of the week follow the same system as the first session. You alternate between lower-body and upper-body exercises in the first half of the session to allow your muscles to recover without giving your heart and lungs a rest. The exercises we've selected are excellent fat-burning moves because they involve big movements and lots of different muscles. The squat, for example, will tone your entire lower body while also burning lots of calories, which will speed up your fat loss efforts. Just as you did in the first session, you finish this session with a dynamic abs move followed by a static abs move so that you challenge your midsection from all angles.

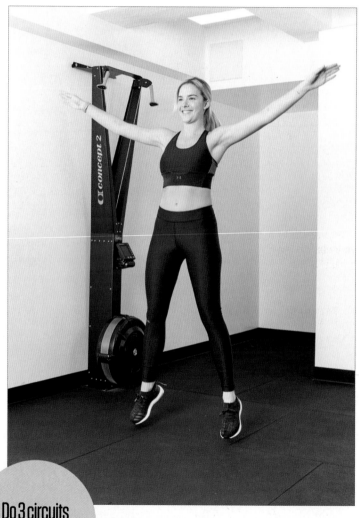

Do 3 circuits in total

EXERCISE	TIME	REST
1 Squat	30sec	30sec
2 Press-up lower	30sec	30sec
3 Reverse lunge	30sec	30sec
4 Star jump	30sec	30sec
5 Bicycle	30sec	30sec
6 Plank	30sec	2min

1 Squat

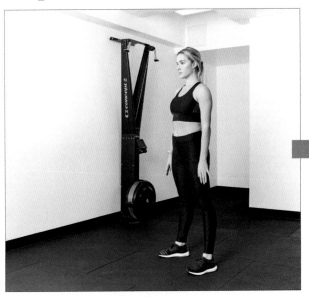

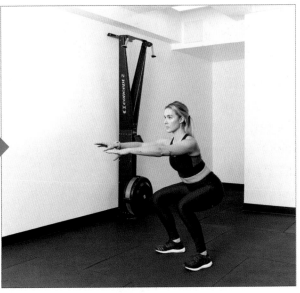

HOW Stand tall, then simultaneously bend at your hips and knees to lower until your thighs are parallel to the floor. Press back up to the start.

WHY This is one of the most effective exercises you can do for toning your bottom and thighs. It will also produce lactic acid, which will help burn fat.

2 Press-up lower

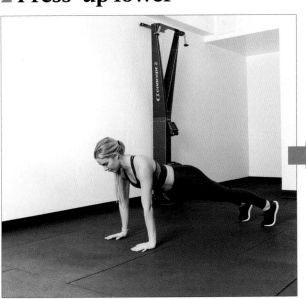

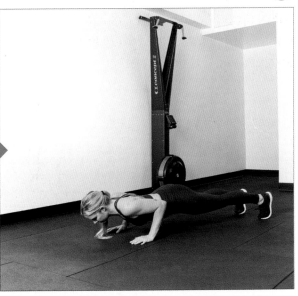

HOW Start at the top of a press-up position, then bend your elbows to lower your body towards the floor. Use your knees to help return to the top and repeat.

WHY You're stronger in the lowering part of this exercise so it's an accessible way of getting the benefits of a full press-up. Make sure you do it in a controlled manner.

3 Reverse lunge

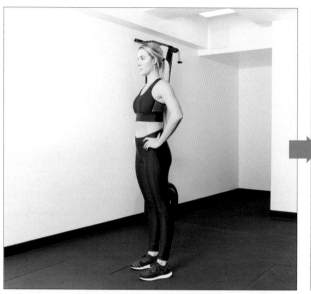 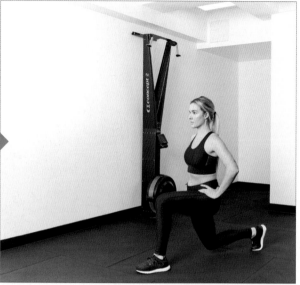

HOW Stand tall, then take a big step backwards and bend your knees until they are both bent at 90 degrees. Push back up to the start and repeat the move on the other side.

WHY The reverse version of the lunge puts more emphasis on your glute muscles and also makes the exercise harder, giving you more of a balance and coordination challenge.

4 Star jump

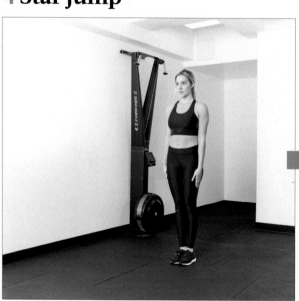 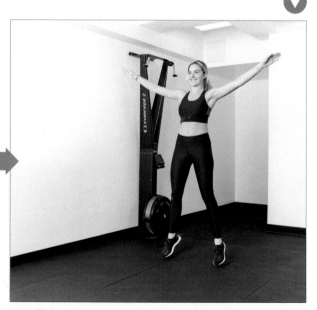

HOW Stand tall, then jump both feet out to the sides while simultaneously raising your arms up in an arc above your head. Jump back to the start and repeat.

WHY This old-school aerobics exercise is worth doing because it is a great way to increase your heart rate quickly without needing much space.

5 Bicycle

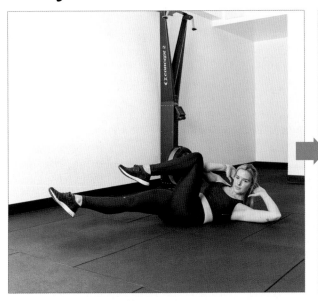
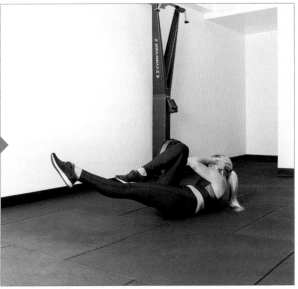

HOW Lie on your back with your hands behind your head. Crunch up to bring one elbow to meet your opposite knee, then repeat on the other side.

WHY This exercise is an excellent way of working your obliques – your side abs. The rotational element of the exercise will also be good for your spinal mobility.

6 Plank

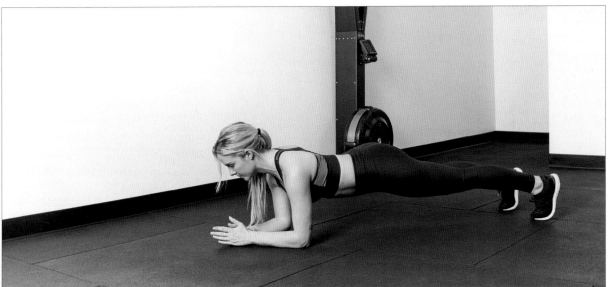

HOW Make sure your body is in a straight line from head to heels. Your elbows should be directly below your shoulders. Hold the position and don't let your hips sag.

WHY The plank is a great way of strengthening the deep-lying core muscles that protect your spine and improve your posture.

Circuit 3

By now you should be getting familiar with the circuit system and this workout follows the same pattern as the first two. The reason that system hasn't changed is two-fold: it's a seriously effective way to exercise, and by repeating the system you get used to exercising in that way. The result is that you're able to work harder during each session because your body gets more familiar with the physical challenge. This workout involves moves like the jump lunge and burpee that will get your heart pounding and help you to sculpt a leaner physique because they encourage you to expend so much energy.

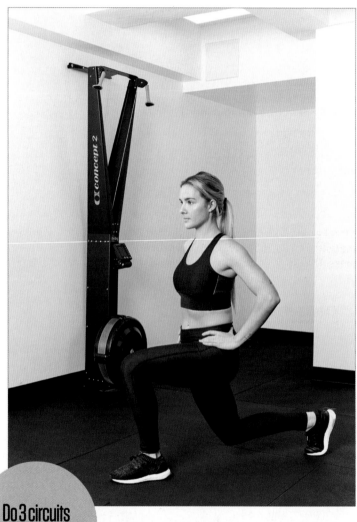

Do 3 circuits in total

EXERCISE	TIME	REST
1 Squat pulse	30sec	30sec
2 Press-up on knees	30sec	30sec
3 Jump lunge	30sec	30sec
4 Burpee	30sec	30sec
5 Russian twist	30sec	30sec
6 Side plank	15sec each side	2min

1 Squat pulse

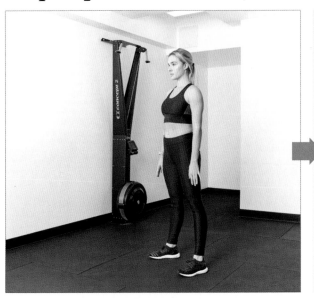

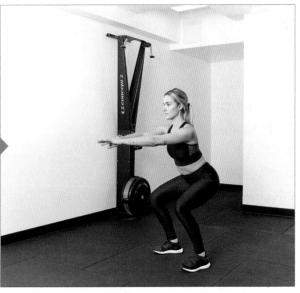

HOW Perform a standard squat and when you reach the bottom of the move, perform a small pulse three times. Then stand up and repeat that pattern.

WHY This version of the move will increase the amount of lactic acid your muscles produce, which has been shown to have a positive effect on fat burning.

2 Press-up on knees

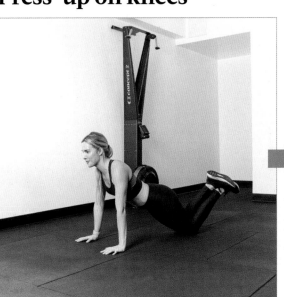

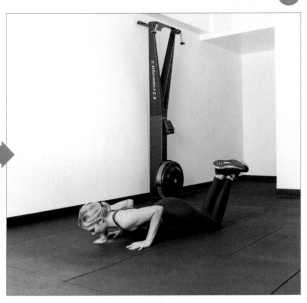

HOW Position yourself so that your arms are straight and your hands are below your shoulders with your body in a straight line from knees to head. Lower and press back up.

WHY This progression towards the full press-up offers similar benefits to the full version but requires less upper body strength.

3 Jump lunge

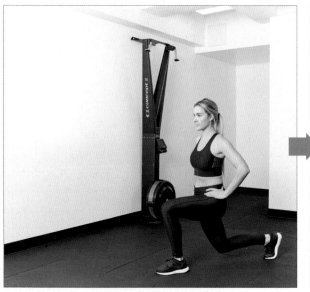 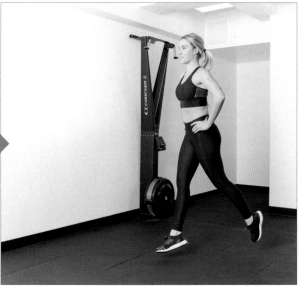

HOW Perform a standard lunge but, instead of returning to the start, jump up explosively and swap legs in mid-air. Land softly and repeat.

WHY This a really tough exercise, which means that you'll be tired at the end of the set but you will also get amazing fat-burning benefits.

4 Burpee

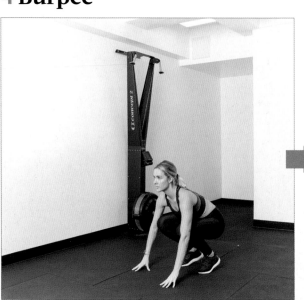 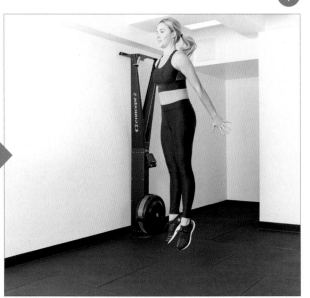

HOW From standing, drop down so your hands are by your feet, jump your feet back then forwards, then jump up with your body upright.

WHY No-one loves doing burpees because they're so tough – but they're one of the most effective exercises you can do if you want to get lean.

5 Russian twist

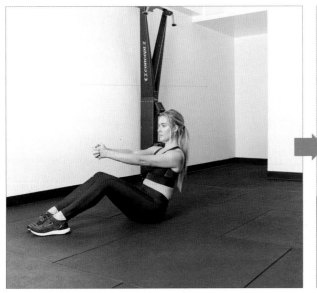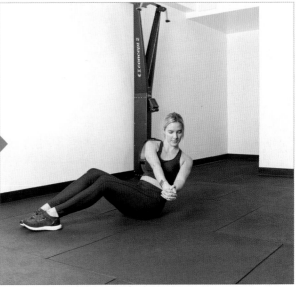

HOW Sit on your bottom with your knees bent and your hands clasped together in front of you. Twist to the left and then twist to the right.

WHY This exercise develops your side abs strength while also challenging your stabilising muscles, which are required to hold your torso upright.

6 Side plank

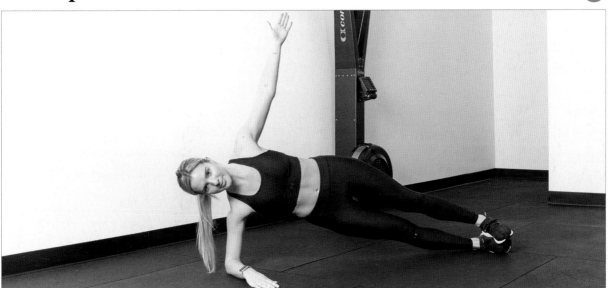

HOW Position yourself on your side, supported on your elbow, then raise your hips and keep your body in a straight line. Hold, then switch to the other side and repeat.

WHY This is another way to work the muscles – specifically the core, abs and lower back, but also the glutes – statically. Doing the side plank also tests your balance.

Circuit 4

The final session of the week is a real challenge. It starts with a tough move – the jump squat – and it doesn't get much easier after that, with a press-up that will test your upper-body strength, a side lunge that will test your balance and coordination, and a tuck jump that will test your explosive power. Work periods of 30 seconds may not sound too long but, trust us, they'll feel a lot longer than that. If you're struggling, remember that quality is better than quantity, so take your time and aim to complete the reps with perfect form.

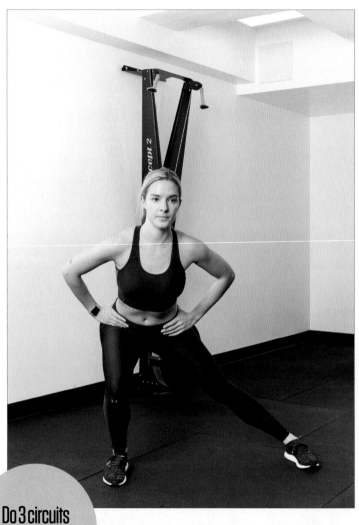

Do 3 circuits in total

EXERCISE	TIME	REST
1 Jump squat	30sec	30sec
2 Press-up	30sec	30sec
3 Side lunge	30sec	30sec
4 Tuck jump	30sec	30sec
5 Crunch	30sec	30sec
6 Plank tap	30sec	2min

1 Squat jump

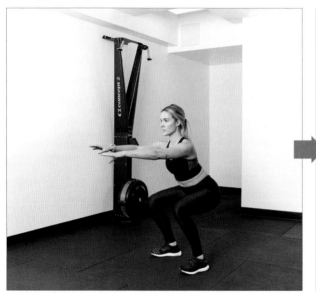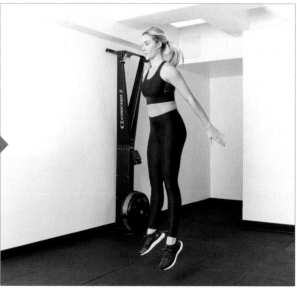

HOW Squat down but, instead of standing back up, jump explosively off the ground. Land softly and repeat the exercise.

WHY Doing a dynamic exercise like this repeatedly without any rest between exercises makes it an intense and highly effective move.

2 Press-up

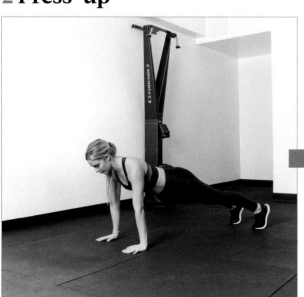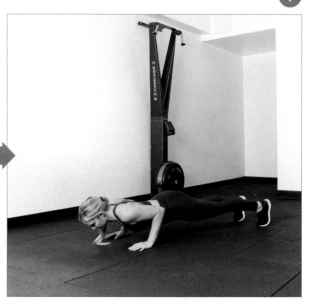

HOW Start with hands below your shoulders with your core and glutes braced. Bend your elbows to lower your chest, then press back up powerfully to return to the start

WHY Press-ups are a very challenging move so don't worry if you can't do many. If you can't do any, just do the lowering portion of the move.

3 Side lunge

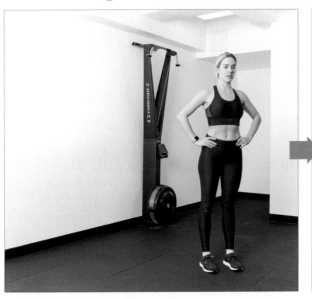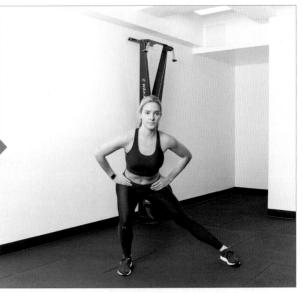

HOW Take a big step to the side and, with both feet pointing forwards, bend your leading knee, keeping your other leg straight. Then return to the start. Alternate sides.

WHY This exercise gives you the same kind of benefits as the lunge while also working your glutes and the insides of your thighs in a different way.

4 Tuck jump

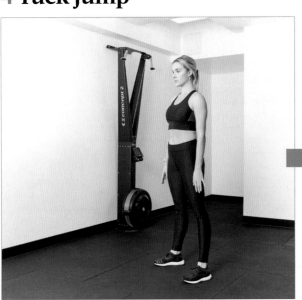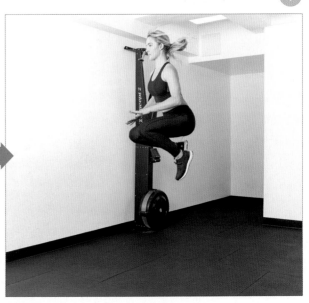

HOW Sink into a quarter squat, then jump up to bring your knees up towards your chest. Land softly, then go straight into the next jump.

WHY This is a good exercise because you can go all-out and give it everything you've got but with very little risk of injury.

5 Crunch

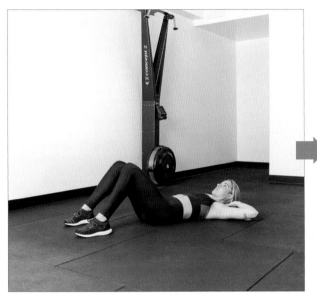 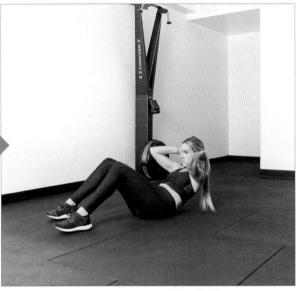

HOW Lie on your back with your knees bent and feet just off the floor. Breathe out, then contract your abs to lift your head and shoulders, then lower.

WHY This is a classic abs exercise but it's only worth doing if you do it properly. Concentrate on really squeezing your abs and performing the exercise slowly.

6 Plank tap

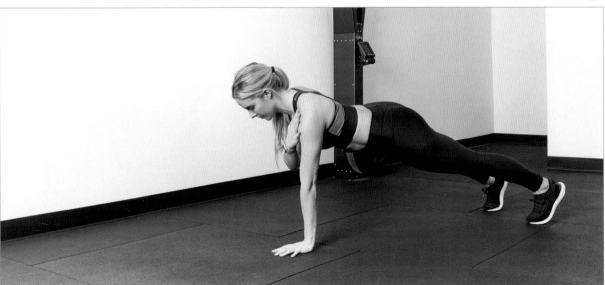

HOW Position yourself in the start of a straight-arm plank. Without rotating your body, touch one hand to your opposite shoulder and repeat the move on the other side.

WHY This gives you the benefits of the plank but also requires you to keep your body stable as you control the urge to twist your torso.

Week 2

Do 4 circuits in total

CIRCUIT 1

EXERCISE	TIME	REST
1 Split squat	30sec	30sec
2 Punches	30sec	30sec
3 Lunge	30sec	30sec
4 Run on the spot	30sec	30sec
5 Mountain climber	30sec	30sec
6 Straight-arm plank	30sec	2min

CIRCUIT 2

EXERCISE	TIME	REST
1 Squat	30sec	30sec
2 Press-up lower	30sec	30sec
3 Reverse lunge	30sec	30sec
4 Star jump	30sec	30sec
5 Bicycle	30sec	30sec
6 Plank	30sec	2min

CIRCUIT 3

EXERCISE	TIME	REST
1 Squat pulse	30sec	30sec
2 Press-up on knees	30sec	30sec
3 Jump lunge	30sec	30sec
4 Burpee	30sec	30sec
5 Russian twist	30sec	30sec
6 Side plank	15sec each side	2min

CIRCUIT 4

EXERCISE	TIME	REST
1 Jump squat	30sec	30sec
2 Press-up	30sec	30sec
3 Side lunge	30sec	30sec
4 Tuck jump	30sec	30sec
5 Crunch	30sec	30sec
6 Plank tap	30sec	2min

Week 3

Do 3 circuits in total

CIRCUIT 1

EXERCISE	TIME	REST
1 Split squat	40sec	20sec
2 Punches	40sec	20sec
3 Lunge	40sec	20sec
4 Run on the spot	40sec	20sec
5 Mountain climber	40sec	20sec
6 Straight-arm plank	40sec	90sec

CIRCUIT 2

EXERCISE	TIME	REST
1 Squat	40sec	20sec
2 Press-up lower	40sec	20sec
3 Reverse lunge	40sec	20sec
4 Star jump	40sec	20sec
5 Bicycle	40sec	20sec
6 Plank	40sec	90sec

CIRCUIT 3

EXERCISE	TIME	REST
1 Squat pulse	40sec	20sec
2 Press-up on knees	40sec	20sec
3 Jump lunge	40sec	20sec
4 Burpee	40sec	20sec
5 Russian twist	40sec	20sec
6 Side plank	20sec each side	90sec

CIRCUIT 4

EXERCISE	TIME	REST
1 Jump squat	40sec	20sec
2 Press-up	40sec	20sec
3 Side lunge	40sec	20sec
4 Tuck jump	40sec	20sec
5 Crunch	40sec	20sec
6 Plank tap	40sec	90sec

Week 4

Do 4 circuits in total

CIRCUIT 1

EXERCISE	TIME	REST
1 Split squat	40sec	20sec
2 Punches	40sec	20sec
3 Lunge	40sec	20sec
4 Run on the spot	40sec	20sec
5 Mountain climber	40sec	20sec
6 Straight-arm plank	40sec	90sec

CIRCUIT 2

EXERCISE	TIME	REST
1 Squat	40sec	20sec
2 Press-up lower	40sec	20sec
3 Reverse lunge	40sec	20sec
4 Star jump	40sec	20sec
5 Bicycle	40sec	20sec
6 Plank	40sec	90sec

CIRCUIT 3

EXERCISE	TIME	REST
1 Squat pulse	40sec	20sec
2 Press-up on knees	40sec	20sec
3 Jump lunge	40sec	20sec
4 Burpee	40sec	20sec
5 Russian twist	40sec	20sec
6 Side plank	20sec each side	90sec

CIRCUIT 4

EXERCISE	TIME	REST
1 Jump squat	40sec	20sec
2 Press-up	40sec	20sec
3 Side lunge	40sec	20sec
4 Tuck jump	40sec	20sec
5 Crunch	40sec	20sec
6 Plank tap	40sec	90sec

Week 5

Do 5 circuits in total

CIRCUIT 1

EXERCISE	REPS/TIME	REST
1 Split squat	40sec	20sec
2 Punches	40sec	20sec
3 Lunge	40sec	20sec
4 Run on the spot	40sec	20sec
5 Mountain climber	40sec	20sec
6 Straight-arm plank	40sec	90sec

CIRCUIT 2

EXERCISE	REPS/TIME	REST
1 Squat	40sec	20sec
2 Press-up lower	40sec	20sec
3 Reverse lunge	40sec	20sec
4 Star jump	40sec	20sec
5 Bicycle	40sec	20sec
6 Plank	40sec	90sec

CIRCUIT 3

EXERCISE	REPS	REST
1 Squat pulse	40sec	20sec
2 Press-up on knees	40sec	20sec
3 Jump lunge	40sec	20sec
4 Burpee	40sec	20sec
5 Russian twist	40sec	20sec
6 Side plank	20sec each side	90sec

CIRCUIT 4

EXERCISE	REPS/TIME	REST
1 Jump squat	40sec	20sec
2 Press-up	40sec	20sec
3 Side lunge	40sec	20sec
4 Tuck jump	40sec	20sec
5 Crunch	40sec	20sec
6 Plank tap	40sec	90sec

Week 6

Do 5 circuits in total

CIRCUIT 1

EXERCISE	REPS/TIME	REST
1 Split squat	40sec	15sec
2 Punches	40sec	15sec
3 Lunge	40sec	15sec
4 Run on the spot	40sec	15sec
5 Mountain climber	40sec	15sec
6 Straight-arm plank	40sec	90sec

CIRCUIT 2

EXERCISE	REPS/TIME	REST
1 Squat	40sec	15sec
2 Press-up lower	40sec	15sec
3 Reverse lunge	40sec	15sec
4 Star jump	40sec	15sec
5 Bicycle	40sec	15sec
6 Plank	40sec	90sec

CIRCUIT 3

EXERCISE	REPS	REST
1 Squat pulse	40sec	15sec
2 Press-up on knees	40sec	15sec
3 Jump lunge	40sec	15sec
4 Burpee	40sec	15sec
5 Russian twist	40sec	15sec
6 Side plank	20sec each side	90sec

CIRCUIT 4

EXERCISE	REPS/TIME	REST
1 Jump squat	40sec	15sec
2 Press-up	40sec	15sec
3 Side lunge	40sec	15sec
4 Tuck jump	40sec	15sec
5 Crunch	40sec	15sec
6 Plank tap	40sec	90sec

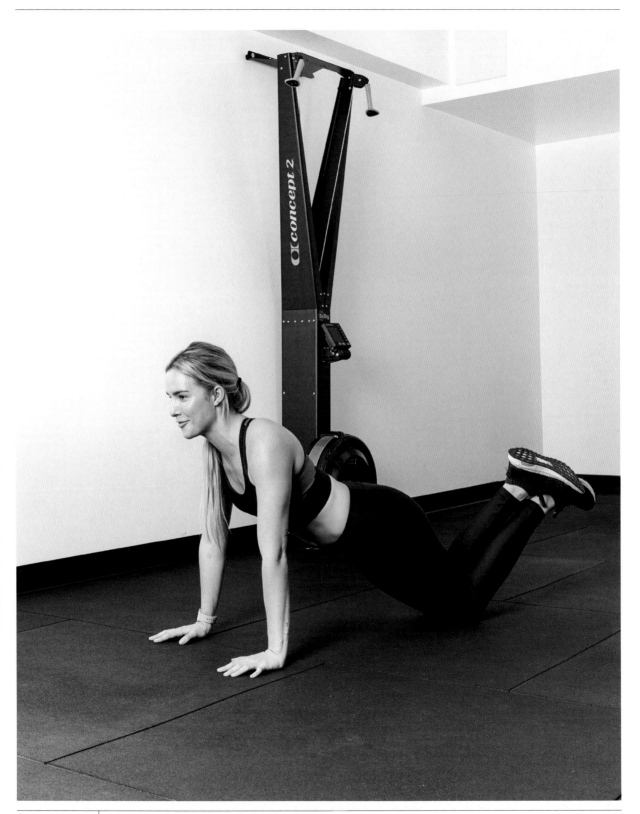

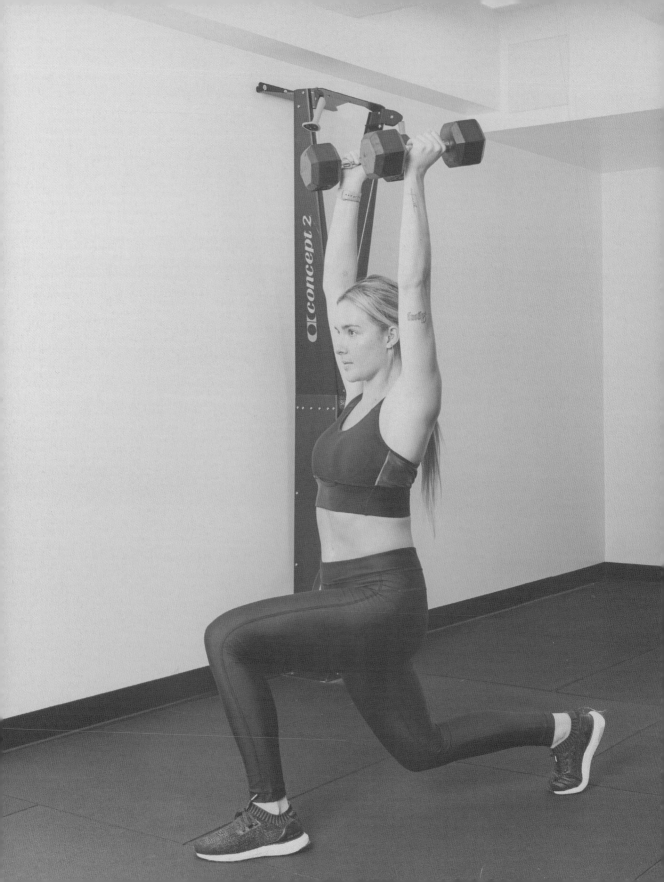

6.

Total body tone-up

Your priority is to burn off body fat, but one of the best ways to do that is to do workouts that tone up your muscles. Why? Not only will you torch fat through training and burn more calories at rest, you'll also sculpt a lean physique and look and feel better than ever! Just use our expert tips and this six-week plan to get started.

In the pursuit of trying to reduce the amount of body fat you carry, it can be easy to get caught in the trap spending more time running and avoiding the foods you love. But as you've learned in the previous chapters, getting lean in the most effective way possible means taking a smarter approach to the way you eat and exercise. And while toning up may not be your priority right now – you want to lose stubborn body fat first and foremost – it will actually make a huge difference to how you look and feel.

Not only do you torch more calories when on the gym floor, but you also burn through more calories in the hours and days after a session as your body recovers from your exertions. Another benefit is that more of the food you eat will be used to meet the demands of your training, so more of the energy and nutrients go towards rebuilding muscle tissue and replenishing glycogen stores rather than being deposited in fat cells, which is what happens when you eat far more than you burn off.

Over the next few pages you'll find all the advice and insight you need to make your resistance-training sessions as effective as possible, which will arm you with all the information you need to train smarter so that you can blitz your belly fast.

We've put together a six-week workout programme that will not only tone up your major muscle groups – specifically your thighs, glutes, arms and abs – to radically transform your physique, but will also place the perfect stimulus on your body to repeatedly tap into its fat stores to use as fuel. The result is that as well as getting leaner and more toned, you'll also get stronger, which will enable you to take on more advanced training approaches once want a new training goal to work towards.

One thing you'll notice is that these resistance training sessions all involve a pair of dumbbells. If you're concerned that lifting weights will make you look bulky, we can dispel that myth right now. It simply won't happen for a couple of reasons. The first is that if you are a woman you don't have the hormonal profile to rapidly add muscle, particularly if you're a relatively inexperienced exerciser. The second is that the plan hasn't been created to add muscle but has been designed to give you a lean, healthy and athletic look.

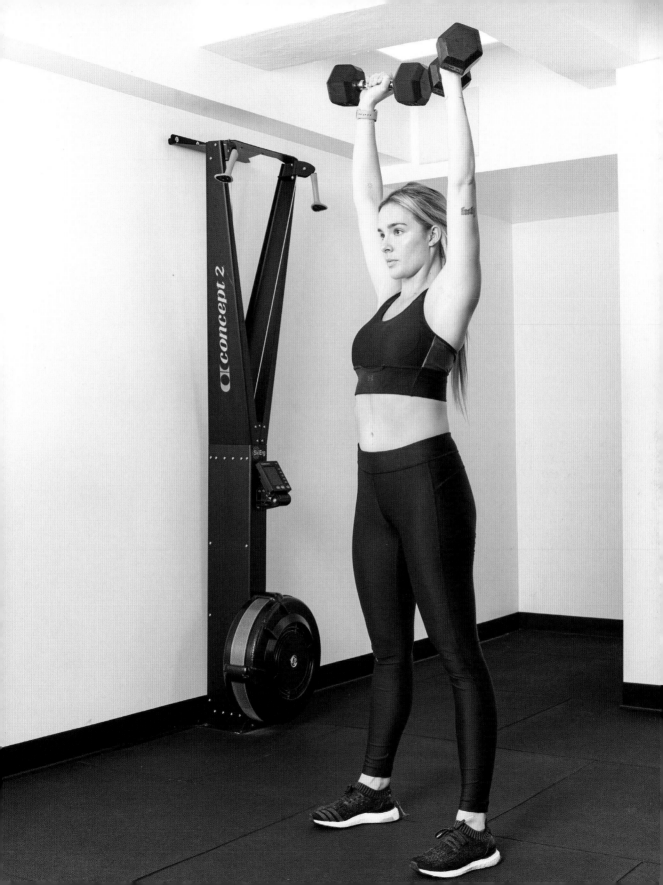

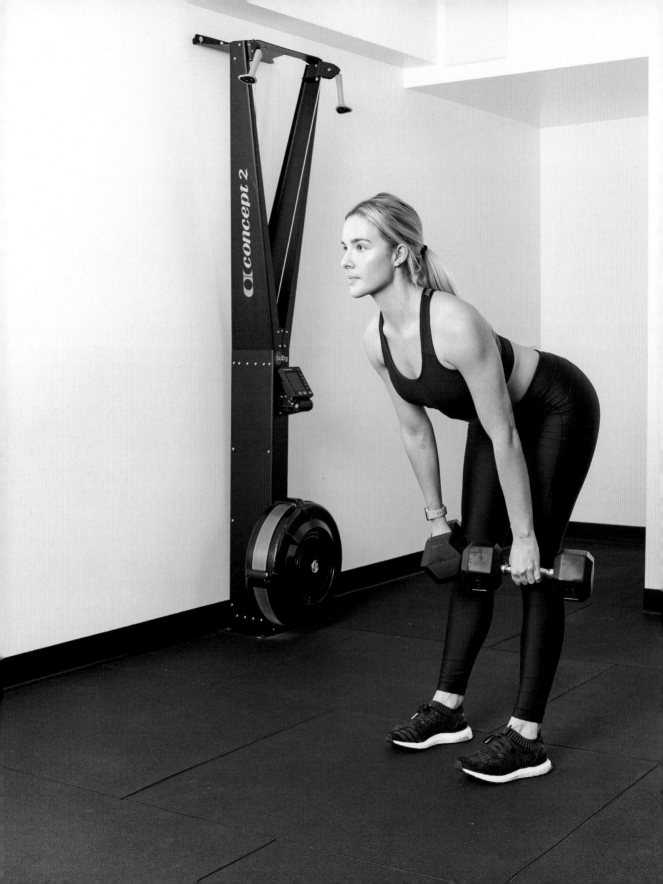

Muscle toning rules

MAINTAIN PERFECT FORM

Before you even think about picking up a dumbbell, make sure you are completely comfortable with how to perform all the exercises that comprise your workout. This is crucial not only to prevent injury, but also to ensure that each rep of every lift hits the target muscle or muscle group efficiently with no wasted effort. That's the key to making big changes to your body fast.

LIFT THE RIGHT WEIGHT

You might think that lifting anything heavier than 5kg will mean that you wake up the next day with big bulging muscles. The reality is that you should lift the heaviest weight with which you can complete all the reps in the set without compromising your form. If you are new to resistance training, it makes sense to pick a weight that you're comfortable with. As you progress, you can select a heavier weight.

CONTROL YOUR MOVEMENT

Tempo, or the speed that you lift and lower a weight for each rep, determines how much tension your muscles must manage, which is one of the biggest factors in determining the benefits you get from resistance workouts. This means it's essential to stick to a slow and controlled tempo for each move, without bouncing the weight around. The exception is jumping moves, which can be done at speed (known as "explosively").

FOCUS ON YOUR MUSCLES

The mind-to-muscle connection is one of the most effective tactics for muscle toning – yet one of the most under-used. All it means is that when you are performing each rep you need to focus on the body part that is working. Actually looking at the body part, either directly or in a mirror, is a great way to focus your mind on connecting to the muscle group to make it work as hard as possible.

IMPROVE YOUR MINDSET

You need to start every session with the mentality that this is going to be the best workout you've ever had. Attacking each set with intent, purpose and positivity goes a long way in pushing you outside of your comfort zone, which is where you need to be if you want to radically transform your body. Shut out any negative thoughts, stick on your headphones and train like your life depends on it.

Toned in 6 weeks

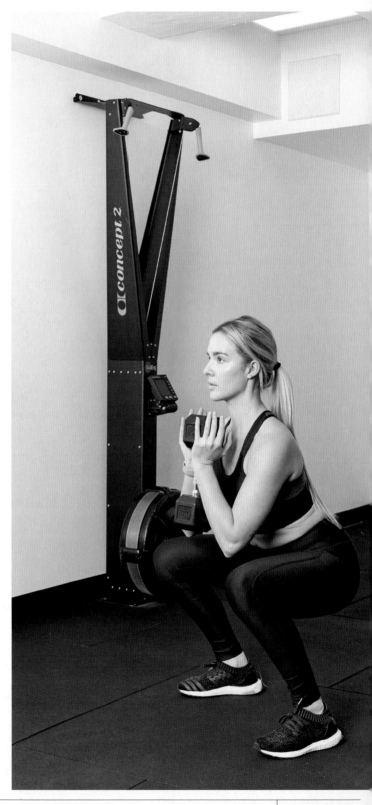

This six-week training programme has been designed so you can tone up while burning excess body fat as quickly as possible. There are four workouts a week, and although the moves you do in each workout remain the same for all six weeks, either the reps per set or sets per workout will increase each week to keep you moving in the right direction. Stick to the exact workout plan so you do the exercises listed in each workout in the order indicated, and keep to the sets, reps and rest periods detailed. By following this plan perfectly, you'll be able to tone up and burn fat to build a stronger and leaner body. Do it right and you might just be amazed by what you achieve.

HOW DOES THIS PLAN WORK?

This six-week workout plan will tone muscle while stripping away fat because it's a progressive programme that pushes you a little further out of your comfort zone every time you train. This approach gives your body no choice but to keep changing and adapting for the better. Always asking your body to work a bit harder is tough, and there'll be times you want to quit, but every session you successfully complete will take you a step closer to a better body.

DO I NEED TO FOLLOW IT EXACTLY?

If you want to get the best results possible you need to follow the plan to the letter. This four-times-a-week training programme has been designed to push your body hard, and chopping and changing will reduce its effectiveness. Consistency is crucial to any successful fat loss challenge so you need to find the time to work out four times a week every week for six weeks, even if that means sacrificing some of your free time. It will be worth it in the end.

WHAT WEIGHT DO I LIFT?

Finding your starting weight for each exercise may need a little trial and error, and it's best to start light if in doubt, then increase the weight in subsequent sets. As a rule you should find the last few reps of a set challenging. If you finish the set and feel like you could have done another five reps, the weight you are lifting is too light; if you only perform half the target reps before your muscles fail, it's too heavy.

WHAT DO I DO AFTER THE PLAN?

The beauty of following this six-week plan is that you'll gain strength as well as toning up and stripping away fat. This will enable you to take your training to the next level once you've completed it. At that point you can focus on a new plan that's in line with your long-term goal. Alternatively you can simply repeat this plan, but your new strength means you will be able to start with heavier weights and keep progressing accordingly.

Warm up to perform better

Performing a short but focused warm-up before a resistance workout is essential to prepare your mind and muscles for the session ahead. Gradually increasing the effort and intensity through your warm-up helps your body go from a rested to an active state by increasing your heart rate to pump more oxygenated blood to your muscles, enabling them to do the heavy lifting that's required to change your body for the better. Just as importantly, a thorough warm-up will reduce your chance of picking up a muscle strain or injury, which is the last thing you want – it's very hard to lose body fat and tone up if you can't work out. Here's what you need to know about performing the perfect warm-up to make every weights session more effective.

THINK DYNAMIC STRETCHES

A lot of research has been carried out on the subject of stretching in recent years and the experts have generally concluded that you should avoid static stretches, where you hold a position for a period of time, pre-workout. Instead, they advise doing dynamic stretches such as squats and lunges without weights. These will prime your body to take on the exercises and physical demands posed by your session.

DO THE FIRST TWO MOVES

Before starting the main workout, you need to warm up by performing the first two moves of the workout. Start with a light weight and do as many reps of both moves as it takes for you to start to feel the muscles working. The aim here is to get blood flowing to your target muscles. You're also warming up your joints to prevent injury and you're aiming to gradually increase your heart rate.

WARM UP YOUR MIND AS WELL

A good warm-up will prepare you physically for a better session by elevating your core body temperature, which makes muscles warmer and more elastic, as well as increasing blood flow to your muscles. But for the best workout possible you need to mentally prepare too. Use your warm-up time to visualise the moves ahead and think about how your muscles will feel. Also think how good you'll feel once you put another successful session in the bag.

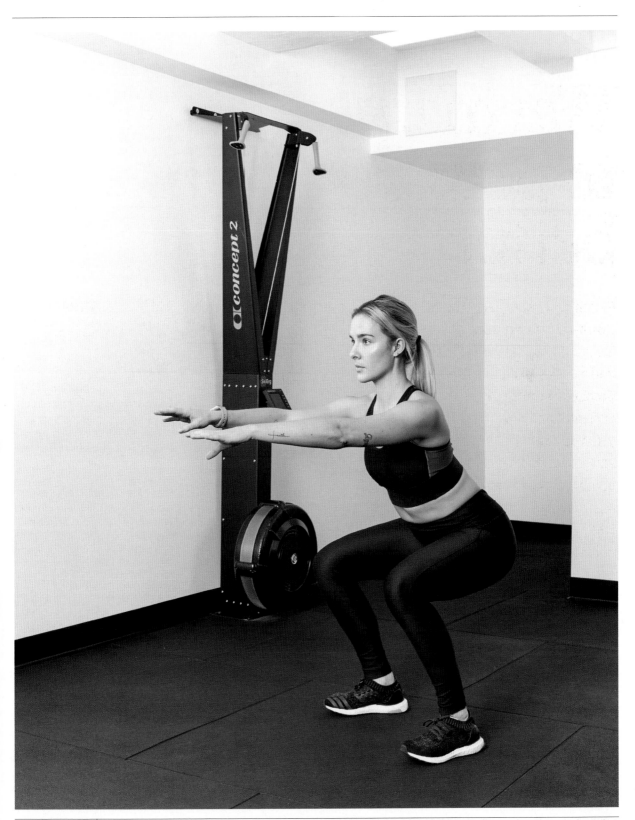

Week 1
Workout 1

Your six-week plan uses the same workout format throughout. It involves doing two supersets at the start of your workout. A superset is two exercises performed back to back with minimal rest, so they are a bit like a mini circuit. The benefit of supersets is that they challenge your muscles and also your cardiovascular system because you don't get any rest. In each superset, we've selected two exercises that work different parts of your body. This makes them more accessible from a muscle challenge point of view (because one muscle works while the other rests) and more demanding from a cardiovascular point of view (because your body has to shuttle oxygen to different areas). The workout finishes with an exercise that targets your glutes and then a move that works your abs in a fun and dynamic way.

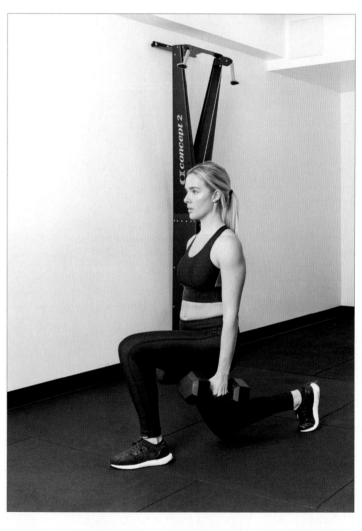

EXERCISE	SETS	REPS	REST
1a Dumbbell squat	2	12	0sec
1b Press-up lower	2	12	60sec
2a Dumbbell lunge	2	6 each side	0sec
2b Overhead press	2	12	60sec
3 Romanian deadlift	2	12	60sec
4 Plank drag	2	8 each side	60sec

1a Dumbbell squat

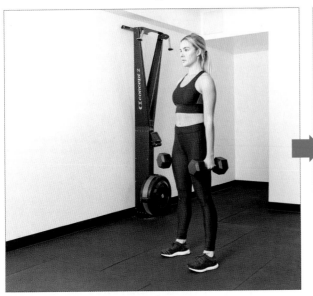

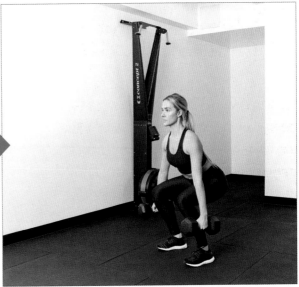

START Stand tall with your chest up and core tight, holding a dumbbell in each hand, keeping your arms straight.

MOVEMENT With your chest up, squat down by bending your knees – keeping them in line with your toes – until your hips are below knee height. Press down through your heels to return to the start position.

1b Press-up lower

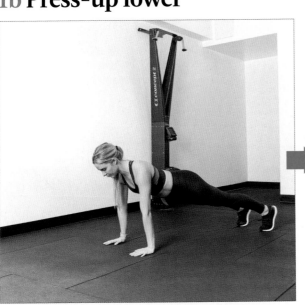

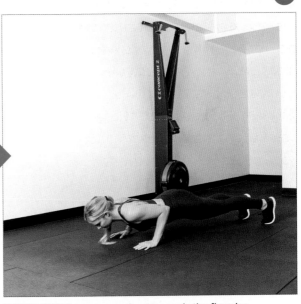

START Position yourself so that your body is straight from head to heels and your arms are straight with your hands directly below your shoulders.

MOVEMENT Lower your chest towards the floor by bending your elbows, keeping them close to your sides. Go onto your knees to press back up.

2a Dumbbell lunge

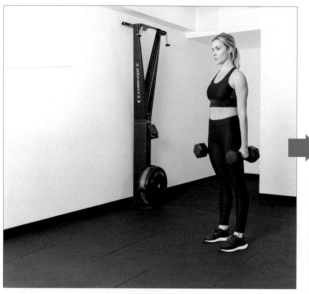

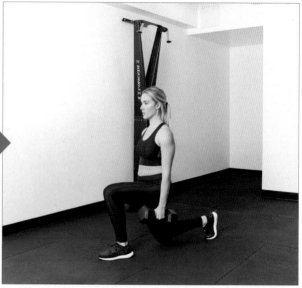

START Stand tall with your chest up and core tight with your feet about hip-width apart.

MOVEMENT Keeping your chest up, take a big step forwards, then lower until both knees are bent at 90 degrees. Push back from your front foot to return to the start. Repeat the move, leading with the other foot. Alternate with each rep.

2b Overhead press

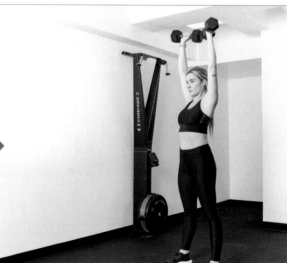

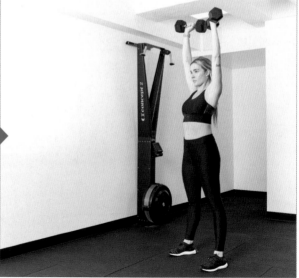

START Stand with your chest up and abs tight, holding a dumbbell in each hand at shoulder height.

MOVEMENT Keeping your chest up, press the weights directly overhead until your arms are straight. Lower them slowly and under control back to the start.

3 Romanian deadlift

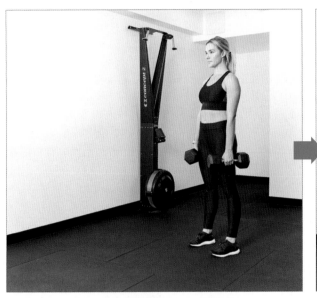
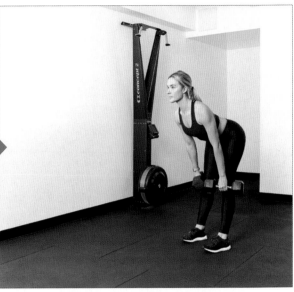

START Stand tall with your chest up and core tight with your feet about hip-width apart and knees slightly bent, holding a dumbbell in each hand.

MOVEMENT Hinge at the hips to push your bottom back and lower the dumbbells down the front of your thighs until you feel a strong stretch, then return to the start.

4 Plank drag

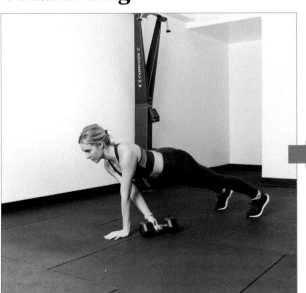
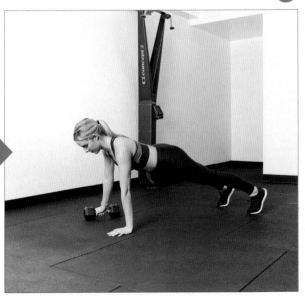

START Start in the top of a press-up so your body is straight from head to heels and your arms are straight. Place a dumbbell to your side.

MOVEMENT Reach under your body to grab the dumbbell with your opposite hand and pull it through to the other side of your body. Repeat using the opposite arm.

Workout 2

The second workout in this first week of the plan follows the same system that you used in the first session. There are two reasons to stick with this system: it's a highly effective way to exercise, and by repeating the system you get used to exercising in that way. The result is that you're able to work harder during each session because your body gets more familiar with the physical challenge. The session is composed of two supersets, an exercise that targets your glutes and a final move that works your midsection dynamically to help sculpt a flat stomach. Remember not to rest after the first move of each superset.

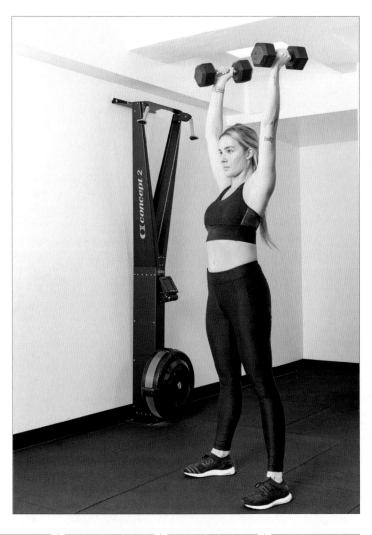

EXERCISE	SETS	REPS	REST
1a Goblet squat	2	12	0sec
1b Elevated press-up	2	12	60sec
2a Dumbbell reverse lunge	2	6 each side	0sec
2b Push press	2	12	60sec
3 One-leg Romanian deadlift	2	6 each side	60sec
4 Russian twist	2	12	60sec

1a Goblet squat

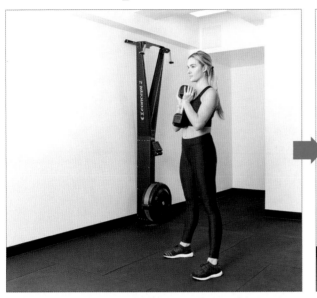

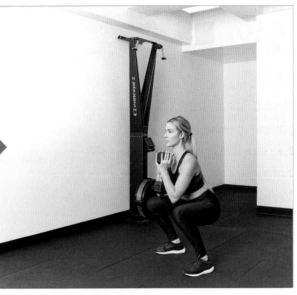

START Stand tall with your chest up and core tight, holding a single dumbbell in both hands at chin height (as if you were about to take a drink from a goblet – hence the name!).

MOVEMENT Keeping your chest up, bend your knees – keeping them in line with your toes – to lower until your hips are below knee height. Press down through your heels to return to the standing position.

1b Elevated press-up

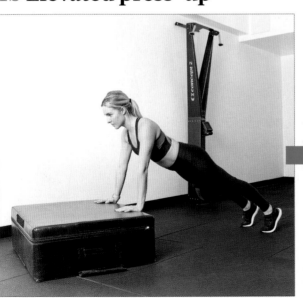

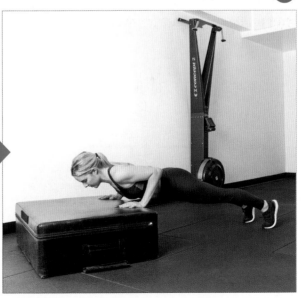

START Position yourself so that your body is straight from head to heels and your arms are straight with your hands directly below your shoulders on a raised platform.

MOVEMENT Lower your chest towards the floor by bending your elbows, keeping them close to your sides, then press back up to the start.

2a Dumbbell reverse lunge

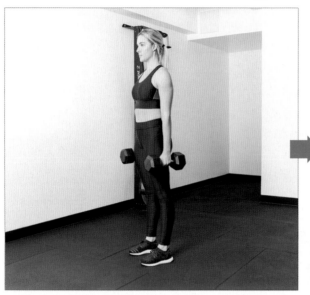

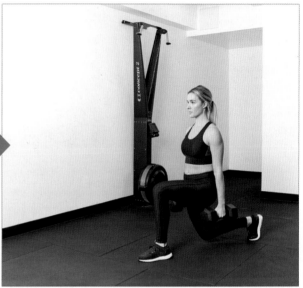

START Stand tall with your chest up and core tight with your feet about hip-width apart, holding a pair of dumbbells.

MOVEMENT Take a big step backwards and simultaneously bend both knees until your back knee is just above the floor. Then press back up to the start. Alternate legs with each rep.

2b Push press

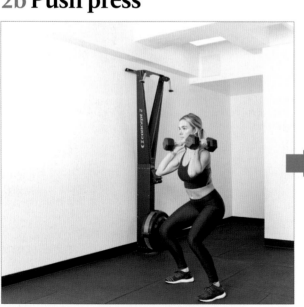

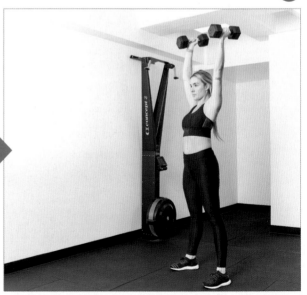

START Stand tall with your chest up and core tight with your feet about hip-width apart, holding a dumbbell in each hand at shoulder height. Bend your knees to lower into a quarter squat.

MOVEMENT Push up and press both weights directly above your head, keeping your wrists below your the weight. Then lower under control back to the quarter squat position.

3 One-leg Romanian deadlift

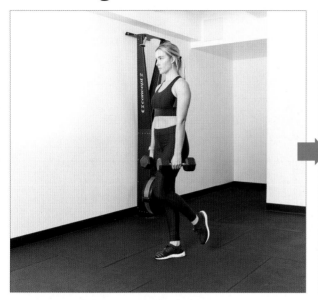

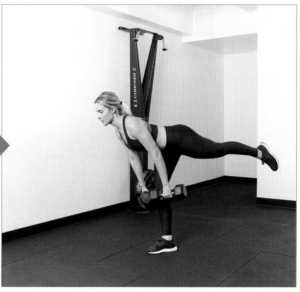

START Stand on one leg with your chest up and abs tight, holding a dumbbell in each hand.

MOVEMENT Keeping your chest up, bend from the hips to lower the weights until you feel a good stretch in the back of that thigh. Reverse the movement back to the start. Complete all the reps on one side, then switch,

4 Russian twist

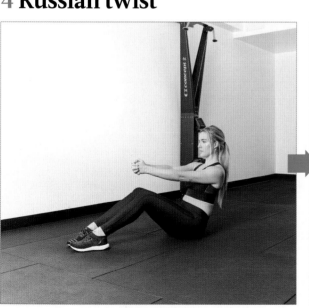

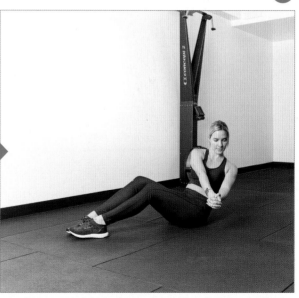

START Lie flat on the floor with knees bent and arms straight and your palms together over your chest. Engage your abs to raise your torso off the floor.

MOVEMENT From this position, rotate your torso to one side, then the other. That's one rep. Keeping your abs tight and your arms straight and palms together throughout.

Workout 3

By now you should be familiar with the workout format and confident about taking on the challenge that each session presents. The first superset in this workout involves one standing exercise and one where you're lying on the floor. Even the act of moving from standing to lying and back again will encourage your heart rate to rise and get blood pumping around your body. The second superset contains a whole-body move that will also test your balance and coordination. As always, the session ends with a glute-sculpting move and a dynamic abs exercise.

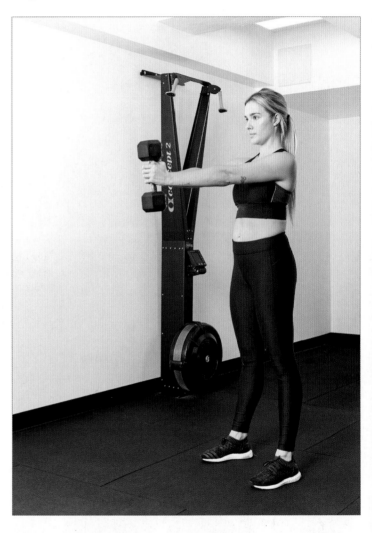

EXERCISE	SETS	REPS	REST
1a Sumo squat	2	12	0sec
1b Dumbbell floor press	2	12	60sec
2a Dumbbell lunge press	2	6 each side	0sec
2b Bent-over row	2	12	60sec
3 Stiff-leg Romanian deadlift	2	12	60sec
4 Standing Russian twist	2	12	60sec

1a Sumo squat

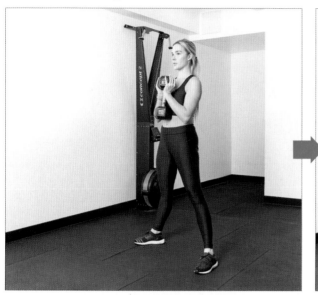

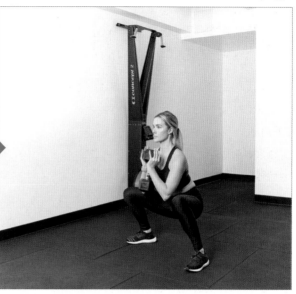

START Stand tall with your chest up and core tight with your feet about twice hip-width apart, holding a dumbbell in both hands at your chest.

MOVEMENT Simultaneously bend at the hips and knees to lower towards the floor until your bottom is level with your knees. Keep your chest up and your weight on your heels. Then press back up to the start.

1b Floor press

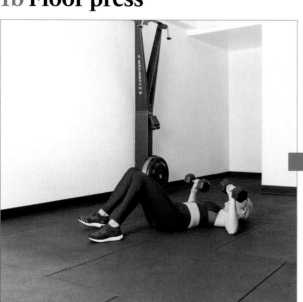

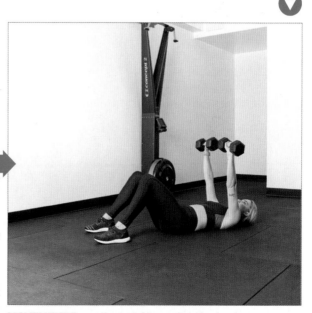

START Lie on the floor with your knees bent at 90 degrees. Hold a dumbbell in each hand with your upper arms on the floor.

MOVEMENT Press the weights up directly above your chest and bring them in to meet in the middle, then lower to the start under control.

2a Dumbbell lunge press

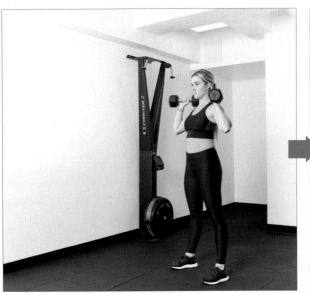

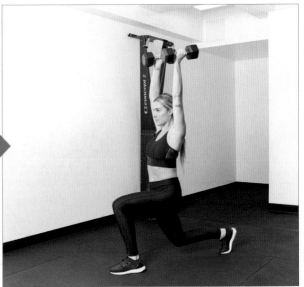

START Stand tall with your chest up, holding a dumbbell in each hand at shoulder height with palms facing away from your body.

MOVEMENT Take a big step forwards, then lower until both knees are bent at 90 degrees. As you lower, press the weights directly overhead.

2b Bent-over row

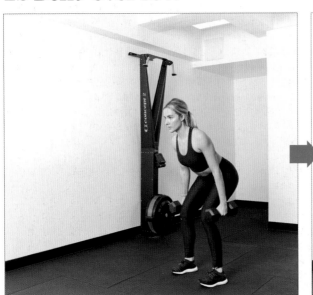

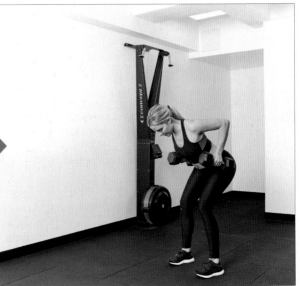

START Stand with your chest up and abs tight, holding a dumbbell in each hand with arms straight. Bend forwards from the hips, keeping your chest up and core tight.

MOVEMENT Leading with your elbows, row the weights up towards your torso. Pause briefly at the top, then lower them back to the start position.

3 Stiff-leg Romanian deadlift

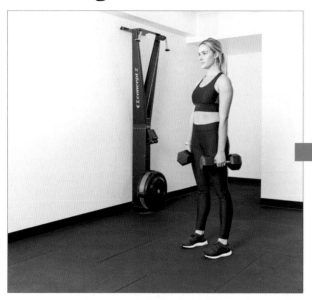 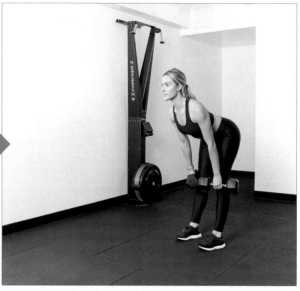

START Stand tall with your chest up and core tight and your feet about hip-width apart, holding a dumbbell in each hand.

MOVEMENT Keeping your legs straight, hinge at the hips and lower the dumbbells down the front of your thighs until you feel a strong stretch. Then return to the start.

4 Standing Russian twist

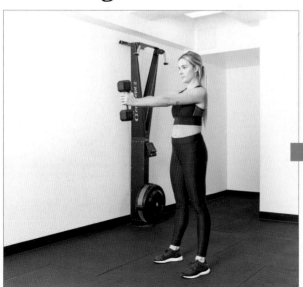 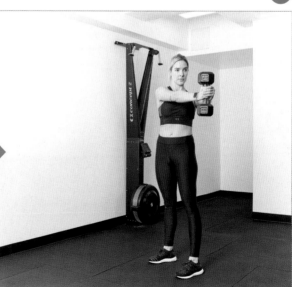

START Stand tall with your chest up and core tight with your feet about hip-width apart, holding a dumbbell in both hands in front of your chest.

MOVEMENT Contract your abs and twist your torso to one side, keeping your arms straight. Twist back to the start and then to the other side and back to complete one rep.

Workout 4

It's the final session of the week and, if you're still going, you should give yourself a pat on the back. Then get down to work and make this the best session of the week. The first superset in this workout involves a fantastic whole-body exercise that will strengthen and tone your thighs and bottom, followed by a fun floor exercise where you "punch" the dumbbells. Whether or not you want to imagine you're punching a particular person is up to you! The penultimate move in the workout, the dumbbell swing, is one of the most useful exercises you can do because it works your posterior chain muscles – the ones on the back of your body that help you stay injury-free and improve your posture.

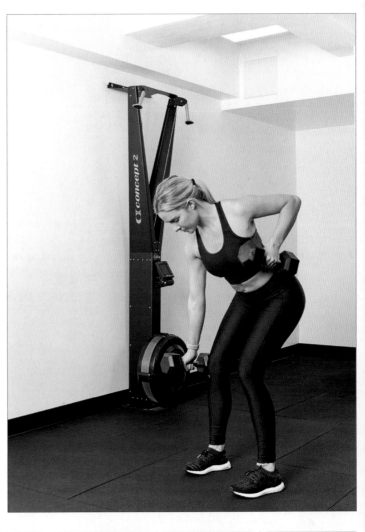

EXERCISE	SETS	REPS	REST
1a Squat press	2	12	0sec
1b Floor punch	2	12	60sec
2a Dumbbell side lunge	2	6 each side	0sec
2b Alternating bent-over row	2	12	60sec
3 Dumbbell swing	2	12	60sec
4 Dumbbell crunch reach	2	12	60sec

1a Squat press

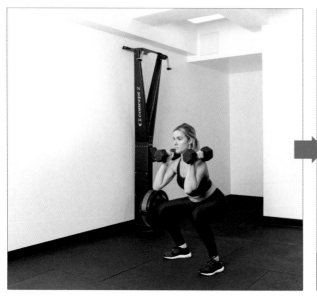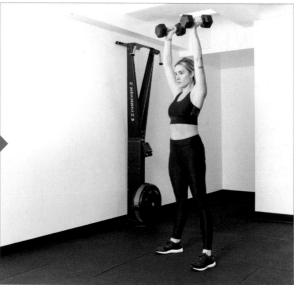

START Stand tall with your chest up and core tight, holding a dumbbell in each hand at shoulder height.

MOVEMENT Keeping your chest up, squat down by bending your knees until your hips are below knee height, while simultaneously pressing the weights directly overhead.

1b Floor punch

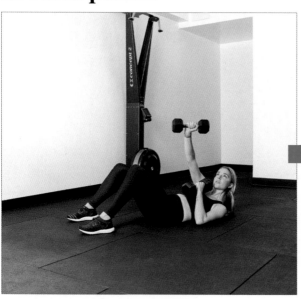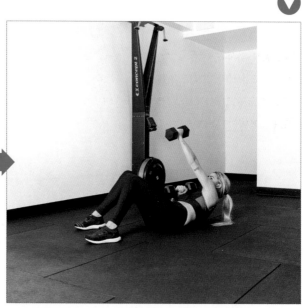

START Lie on the floor with your knees bent at 90 degrees. Hold a dumbbell in each hand with your upper arms on the floor.

MOVEMENT Punch one dumbbell up while raising your shoulder on that side off the floor. As you lower that arm, punch up with the other arm. Lower it to complete one rep and continue alternating.

2a Dumbbell side lunge

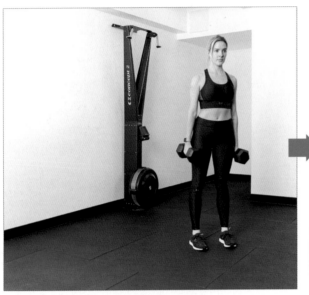
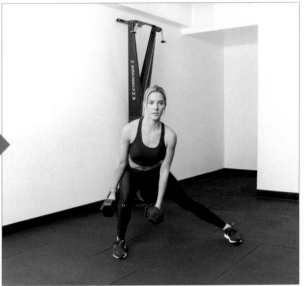

START Stand with your chest up and abs tight with feet hip-width apart. Hold a dumbbell in each hand, keeping your arms straight.

MOVEMENT Keeping your chest up, take a big step to the side, then lower your body as far as you can. Push back off that foot to return to the start then repeat the movement, leading with your other leg. Alternate legs.

2b Alternating bent-over row

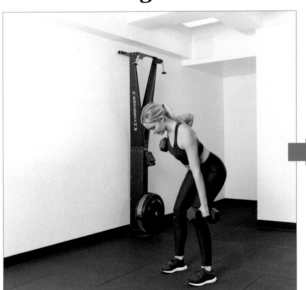
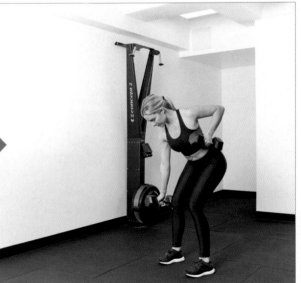

START Stand with your chest up and abs tight holding a dumbbell in each hand with arms straight. Bend forwards from the hips while keeping your chest up and core tight.

MOVEMENT Leading with your elbow, row one weight up towards your torso. Lower them back to the start then repeat the move on the other side to complete one rep.

3 Dumbbell swing

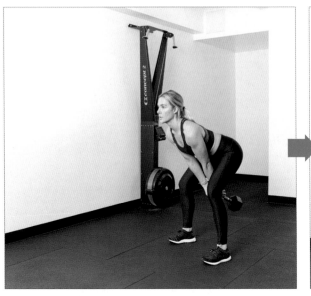

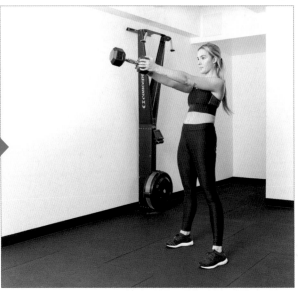

START Stand with your chest up and abs tight with your feet hip-width apart. Hold a dumbbell in both hands between your legs.

MOVEMENT Hinge at the hips to swing the dumbbell back between your legs, then explosively straighten up to bring your hips forwards and the dumbbell up to shoulder height.

4 Dumbbell crunch reach

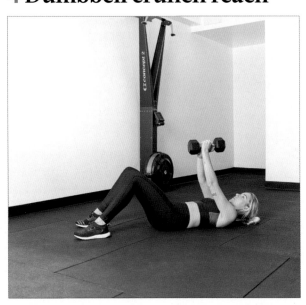

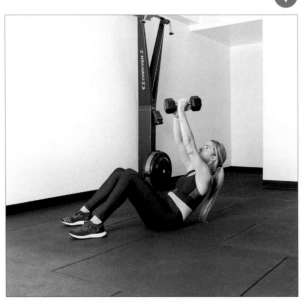

START Lie on your back with your knees bent at 90 degrees. Hold a dumbbell with straight arms above your chest.

MOVEMENT Contract your abs to raise your head and shoulders off the floor while keeping your arms straight and vertical.

Week 2

Workout 1

EXERCISE	SETS	REPS	REST
1a Dumbbell squat	2	15	0sec
1b Press-up lower	2	15	60sec
2a Dumbbell lunge	2	8 each side	0sec
2b Overhead press	2	15	60sec
3 Romanian deadlift	2	15	60sec
4 Plank drag	2	8 each side	60sec

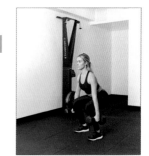

Workout 2

EXERCISE	SETS	REPS	REST
1a Goblet squat	2	15	0sec
1b Elevated press-up	2	15	60sec
2a Dumbbell reverse lunge	2	8 each side	0sec
2b Push press	2	15	60sec
3 One-leg Romanian deadlift	2	8 each side	60sec
4 Russian twist	2	15	60sec

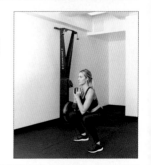

Workout 3

EXERCISE	SETS	REPS	REST
1a Sumo squat	2	15	0sec
1b Dumbbell floor press	2	15	60sec
2a Dumbbell lunge press	2	8 each side	0sec
2b Bent-over row	2	15	60sec
3 Stiff-leg Romanian deadlift	2	15	60sec
4 Standing Russian twist	2	15	60sec

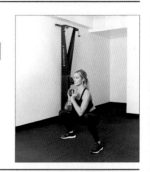

Workout 4

EXERCISE	SETS	REPS	REST
1a Squat press	2	15	0sec
1b Floor punch	2	15	60sec
2a Dumbbell side lunge	2	8 each side	0sec
2b Alternating bent-over row	2	15	60sec
3 Dumbbell swing	2	15	60sec
4 Dumbbell crunch reach	2	15	60sec

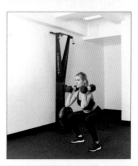

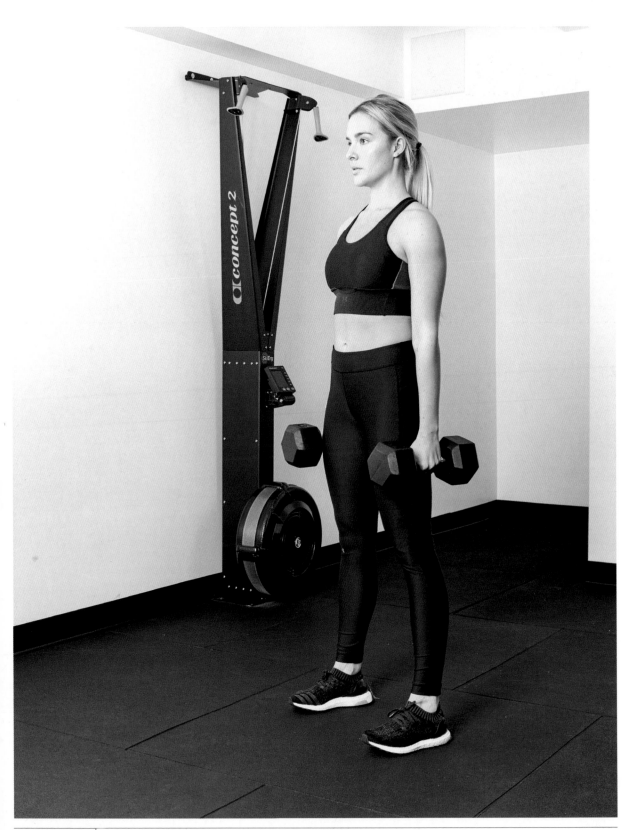

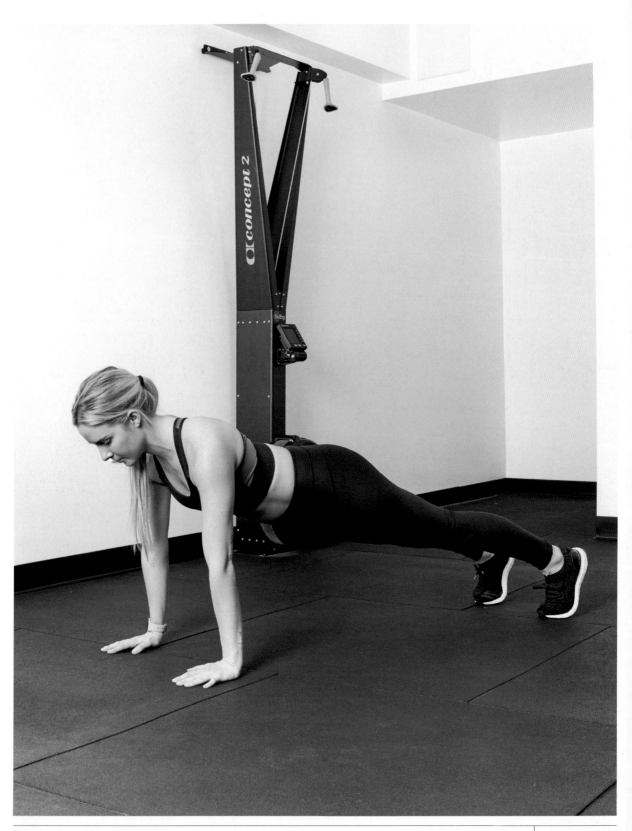

Week 3

Workout 1

EXERCISE	SETS	REPS	REST
1a Dumbbell squat	3	12	0sec
1b Press-up lower	3	12	60sec
2a Dumbbell lunge	3	6 each side	0sec
2b Overhead press	3	12	60sec
3 Romanian deadlift	3	12	60sec
4 Plank drag	3	8 each side	60sec

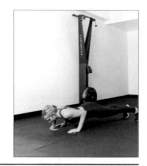

Workout 2

EXERCISE	SETS	REPS	REST
1a Goblet squat	3	12	0sec
1b Elevated press-up	3	12	60sec
2a Dumbbell reverse lunge	3	6 each side	0sec
2b Push press	3	12	60sec
3 One-leg Romanian deadlift	3	6 each side	60sec
4 Russian twist	3	12	60sec

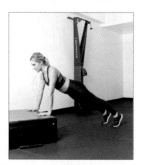

Workout 3

EXERCISE	SETS	REPS	REST
1a Sumo squat	3	12	0sec
1b Dumbbell floor press	3	12	60sec
2a Dumbbell lunge press	3	6 each side	0sec
2b Bent-over row	3	12	60sec
3 Stiff-leg Romanian deadlift	3	12	60sec
4 Standing Russian twist	3	12	60sec

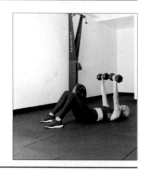

Workout 4

EXERCISE	SETS	REPS	REST
1a Squat press	3	12	0sec
1b Floor punch	3	12	60sec
2a Dumbbell side lunge	3	6 each side	0sec
2b Alternating bent-over row	3	12	60sec
3 Dumbbell swing	3	12	60sec
4 Dumbbell crunch reach	3	12	60sec

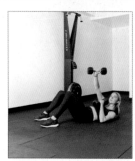

Week 4

Workout 1

EXERCISE	SETS	REPS	REST
1a Dumbbell squat	3	15	0sec
1b Press-up lower	3	15	60sec
2a Dumbbell lunge	3	8 each side	0sec
2b Overhead press	3	15	60sec
3 Romanian deadlift	3	15	60sec
4 Plank drag	3	8 each side	60sec

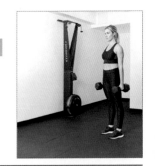

Workout 2

EXERCISE	SETS	REPS	REST
1a Goblet squat	3	15	0sec
1b Elevated press-up	3	15	60sec
2a Dumbbell reverse lunge	3	8 each side	0sec
2b Push press	3	15	60sec
3 One-leg Romanian deadlift	3	8 each side	60sec
4 Russian twist	3	15	60sec

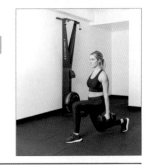

Workout 3

EXERCISE	SETS	REPS	REST
1a Sumo squat	3	15	0sec
1b Dumbbell floor press	3	15	60sec
2a Dumbbell lunge press	3	8 each side	0sec
2b Bent-over row	3	15	60sec
3 Stiff-leg Romanian deadlift	3	15	60sec
4 Standing Russian twist	3	15	60sec

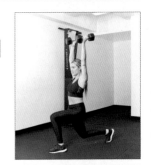

Workout 4

EXERCISE	SETS	REPS	REST
1a Squat press	3	15	0sec
1b Floor punch	3	15	60sec
2a Dumbbell side lunge	3	8 each side	0sec
2b Alternating bent-over row	3	15	60sec
3 Dumbbell swing	3	15	60sec
4 Dumbbell crunch reach	3	15	60sec

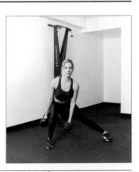

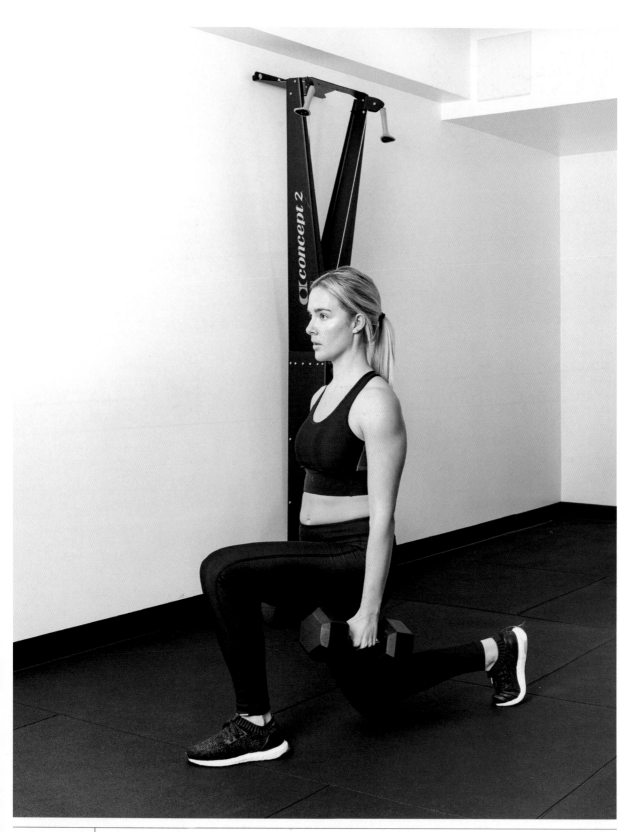

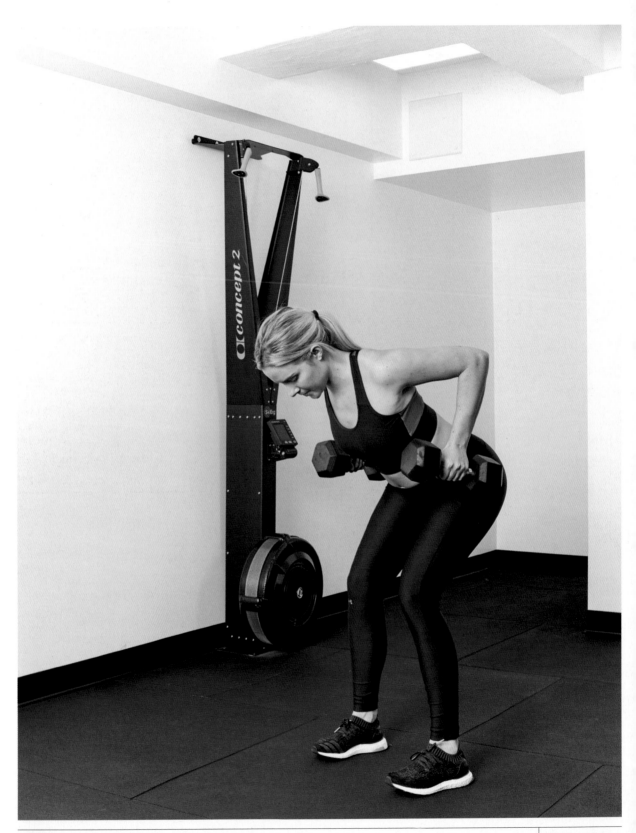

Week 5

Workout 1

EXERCISE	SETS	REPS	REST
1a Dumbbell squat	4	12	0sec
1b Press-up lower	4	12	60sec
2a Dumbbell lunge	4	6 each side	0sec
2b Overhead press	4	12	60sec
3 Romanian deadlift	4	12	60sec
4 Plank drag	4	8 each side	60sec

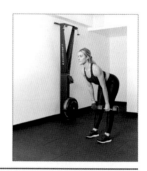

Workout 2

EXERCISE	SETS	REPS	REST
1a Goblet squat	4	12	0sec
1b Elevated press-up	4	12	60sec
2a Dumbbell reverse lunge	4	6 each side	0sec
2b Push press	4	12	60sec
3 One-leg Romanian deadlift	4	6 each side	60sec
4 Russian twist	4	12	60sec

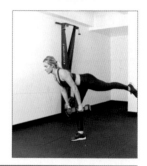

Workout 3

EXERCISE	SETS	REPS	REST
1a Sumo squat	4	12	0sec
1b Dumbbell floor press	4	12	60sec
2a Dumbbell lunge press	4	6 each side	0sec
2b Bent-over row	4	12	60sec
3 Stiff-leg Romanian deadlift	4	12	60sec
4 Standing Russian twist	4	12	60sec

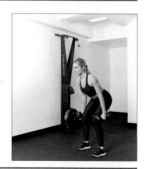

Workout 4

EXERCISE	SETS	REPS	REST
1a Squat press	4	12	0sec
1b Floor punch	4	12	60sec
2a Dumbbell side lunge	4	6 each side	0sec
2b Alternating bent-over row	4	12	60sec
3 Dumbbell swing	4	12	60sec
4 Dumbbell crunch reach	4	12	60sec

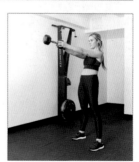

Week 6

Workout 1

EXERCISE	SETS	REPS	REST
1a Dumbbell squat	4	15	0sec
1b Press-up lower	4	15	60sec
2a Dumbbell lunge	4	8 each side	0sec
2b Overhead press	4	15	60sec
3 Romanian deadlift	4	15	60sec
4 Plank drag	4	8 each side	60sec

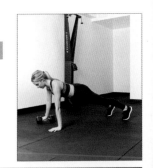

Workout 2

EXERCISE	SETS	REPS	REST
1a Goblet squat	4	15	0sec
1b Elevated press-up	4	15	60sec
2a Dumbbell reverse lunge	4	8 each side	0sec
2b Push press	4	15	60sec
3 One-leg Romanian deadlift	4	8 each side	60sec
4 Russian twist	4	15	60sec

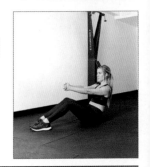

Workout 3

EXERCISE	SETS	REPS	REST
1a Sumo squat	4	15	0sec
1b Dumbbell floor press	4	15	60sec
2a Dumbbell lunge press	4	8 each side	0sec
2b Bent-over row	4	15	60sec
3 Stiff-leg Romanian deadlift	4	15	60sec
4 Standing Russian twist	4	15	60sec

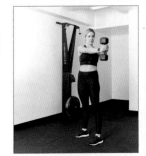

Workout 4

EXERCISE	SETS	REPS	REST
1a Squat press	4	15	0sec
1b Floor punch	4	15	60sec
2a Dumbbell side lunge	4	8 each side	0sec
2b Alternating bent-over row	4	15	60sec
3 Dumbbell swing	4	15	60sec
4 Dumbbell crunch reach	4	15	60sec

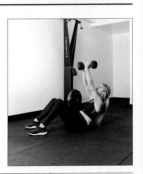